HERBS

PLAIN & SIMPLE

OVER 100 RECIPES FOR HEALTH AND HEALING

Marlene Houghton, PhD

THE ONLY BOOK YOU'LL EVER NEED

HAMPTON ROADS

Cover design by Jim Warner
Interior design by Kathryn Sky-Peck
The image on page 5 comes from Wellcome Images, a website operated by Wellcome Trust, a
global charitable foundation based in the United Kingdom. [wellcomeimages.org]

Hampton Roads Publishing Company, Inc.
Charlottesville, VA 22906
Distributed by Red Wheel/Weiser, LLC
www.redwheelweiser.com
Sign up for our newsletter and special offers by going to
www.redwheelweiser.com/newsletter/

*The author and publisher are not responsible for any adverse effects or consequences resulting from
the use of any remedies, procedures, or preparations included herein.*
*No responsibility is taken for the use of any herb, and although all of the herbs mentioned are
understood to be safe, they should be taken as directed and prescribed by a qualified medical herbalist.*

ISBN: 978-1-57174-766-2

Library of Congress Cataloging-in-Publication Data available upon request

Printed in Canada
MAR
10 9 8 7 6 5 4 3 2 1

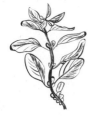

Contents

Introduction. iv

Part One: Herbs and Health

1   A History of Herbalism. 3

2   Herbal Healing. 11

3   Active Properties of Herbs 17

4   A Green Pharmacy. 27

Part Two: Herbs for Different Body Systems

5   Using Herbs to Heal the Body. 35

6   The Immune System 39

7   The Heart and Circulatory System 49

8   The Digestive System. 57

9   The Endocrine System 65

10   The Lymphatic System 75

11   The Muscular System 81

12   The Nervous System. 87

13   The Respiratory System 97

14   The Reproductive System 105

15   The Skeletal System 113

16   The Skin and Eyes 121

17   The Urinary System. 127

Part Three: Herbs for Everyday Use

18   Herbal First Aid Kit 133

19   Health from the Hive 137

20   Herbal Elixirs 147

21   Anti-Aging and Tonic Herbs. 151

22   Aromatic Herbal Baths. 159

23   Herbal Teas. 165

Introduction

There have been many books written on herbal medicine. My book differs from most because it is based on the empowerment model, which focuses on helping people to take responsibility for their own health. This book will help you tackle everyday ailments by taking the guesswork out of which herbs to use to keep you feeling well. Herbal medicine is useful for a range of common complaints, and gentle and effective herbs can offer benefit where conventional medicine sometimes fails.

In a world where we have become more illness and disease focused, and where insurance can be costly, it is clearly becoming important for individuals to become knowledgeable regarding natural therapies, and to take their health into their own hands. The emphasis here is placed on prevention rather than cure. The use of traditional herbalism can help you attain and maintain a high level of well-being. I hope my book will stimulate your interest in the use of natural therapies for home use, and encourage you to research herbalism further.

In *Herbs Plain and Simple* I discuss the herbs in context of the body system they benefit—herbs for circulation, herbs for the respiratory system, and so forth. I tell you a little about each herb's history, and follow this with the medicinal benefits and how it can be used. You will see that many herbs can be used to help the same conditions, because they do not contain just one active property, but several substances. You will therefore find some herbs recommended for more than one ailment, because a single herb can have a diversity of health benefits.

Disclaimer

The statements in this book are based on my studies, experience, and personal research into traditional herbal lore, undertaken over many years. Although I hold a doctorate degree in nutrition, **I am not a medical doctor**. My expertise is in nutrition and traditional herbalism.

The information in this book is intended for educational purposes only and not as medical advice. The information in this book is not intended to diagnose, treat, cure, or prevent any disease, nor to provide individual recommendations. Not all herbal remedies mentioned in this book have been scientifically evaluated, and the information provided is based on traditional herbalism and use. The information should not be considered as medical advice, as it is for general information only; the health claims for each herb are anecdotal, and should be used as a guide only. Consultation with a professional herbalist or a medical doctor is recommended for any health problem.

Although all of the herbs mentioned are understood to be safe, they should be taken as directed and prescribed by a qualified medical herbalist. Herbal remedies come in various forms: tablets, capsules, tinctures, and teas. Please note that some herbs and essential oils may now only be available from qualified medical herbalists.

Warning: Pregnant women should not take any herbs or use any aromatherapy oil without consulting a medical doctor. The same applies for anyone with a serious medical condition or on medication.

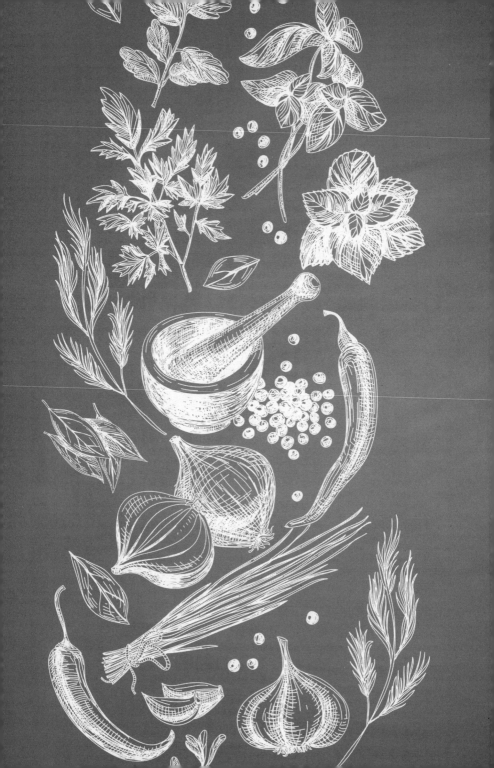

Part One

HERBS
AND
HEALTH

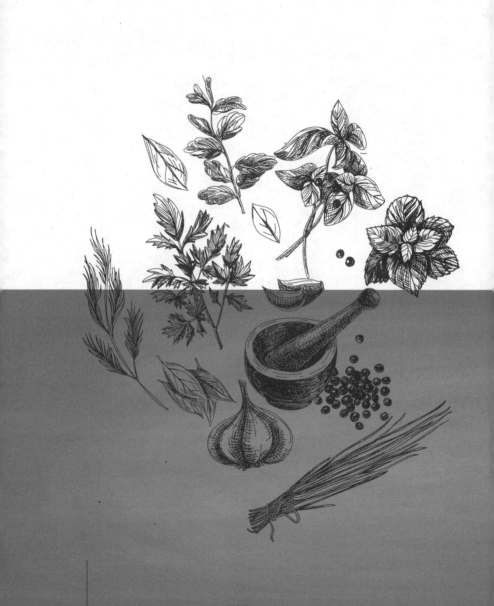

A History
of Herbalism

1

"A weed is a plant whose virtue
is not yet known."
—Ralph Waldo Emerson

Flowers, barks, and roots have been used for their therapeutic properties in the treatment of disease as far back as the time of the ancient Sumerians. Simply put, for thousands of years, plants have shown their efficiency as natural healers, and traditional herbal medicine can rightly be called "The People's Medicine." Herbalism is the oldest form of medical therapy in the world. It has no starting point in history, and no culture or country can claim ownership. It just evolved; therefore it can be called a universal medicine. Before the advent of modern medicine, people routinely used plant power to maintain their health and ensure their survival, and herbalism is still in use today in many parts of the world. According to the World Health Organization, there are still around eighty percent of people worldwide who rely on plant medicines to treat and cure disease.

The early history of traditional herbalism and medical botany in the Americas dates back to the early native peoples; in the United Kingdom we know it dates back to the time of the Druids, who used the simple herbs of the fields, woods, and meadows to cure various human ailments. They believed that the benefits of healing plants were governed by the sun, moon, and the stars, and that the remedies were prepared for mankind by nature herself.

Archeological evidence shows us that early man had an array of herbal cures, and it is from their ancient sacred texts and "herbals" that many modern medicines have developed, just like modern chemistry, which has its roots in alchemy. The high priest/physicians of Ancient Egypt had a sophisticated knowledge of healing methods, and the *Ebers Papyrus*, a seventy-foot long parchment written in 1500 BC, contains references to more than seven hundred herbal remedies. Evidence of medicinal herbs was excavated

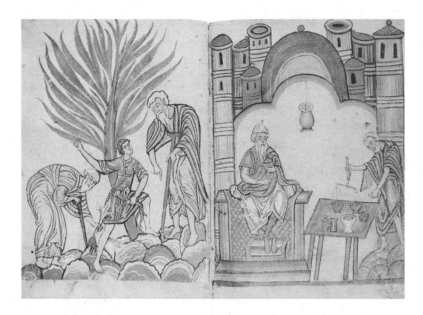

in 1960 in Northern Iraq in a burial ground dating back thousands of years, and it is amazing that many of these herbal remedies are still in use today, proving that their efficacy has withstood the test of time.

Today we are using the wisdom of the ages when we turn to herbs and plants for our health and well-being. By making a connection with the world of nature we are moving toward a more holistic approach to health care and we are returning to our roots. We have inherited this understanding from a time when no man-made drugs were produced and when drug companies did not obtain the active ingredients, extract them, and then sell them in a marketable form. Herbal knowledge of healing has been built on the successful experience of working in harmony with nature, and today there is a growing awareness that to be healthy we have to make healthy choices and to live within nature's laws.

We have begun to grasp the fact that most minor or major illnesses don't just happen out of the blue or because of bad luck. They are the body's reaction to poor living habits and lifestyle choices. Sometimes there are genetic factors, but we are not under the tyranny of our genes as much as was once believed. With their gentle but profound action, herbal remedies are the ideal solution for many common afflictions such as colds, flu, irritable bowel syndrome, insomnia, and stress.

Much herbal wisdom was lost during the witch hunts of the 17th century, which meant that knowledge of natural medicine went underground, but a useful body of herbal knowledge survived. Medicine advanced and herbalism took a back seat until the New Age era of the 1970s, when people began to reconsider the idea of living within nature. A rebirth in the use of plant medicines has seen people take back their power—and take control of their own health. Pharmaceutical medicine just cannot deal with every demand that is made upon it, and in some areas, society has outstripped its ability to pay for everything that is needed.

Despite continuing disregard from the medical world, herbs have always had a part to play. The pharmaceutical drug digitalis is derived from the foxglove plant, and is used in the treatment of heart problems. Two successful cancer treatments, Vincristine and Vinblastine, are derived from the rosy periwinkle shrub, which is native to Southern Madagascar, and these alone have saved the lives of many children with leukemia. How many other plants are waiting to be discovered to be used therapeutically? I would say many, since Mother Nature has not yielded up her many secrets and if these are explored many more healing plants may be discovered.

The ancient herb doctors had sophisticated medical theories of how the human body worked, and they developed a complex set of ideas for the use of medicinal plants. Based on a different philosophical system of hot and cold, herbalists would use hot herbs to treat what was deemed a cold condition and cold herbal compounds in order to cool a system down. In traditional Chinese medicine, this concept of hot and cold herbs is still used. Ayurveda is a traditional Indian healing system that is based on a similar philosophy, where herbal remedies are used to reinstate balance in a system that has lost its equilibrium. The theory of cold or hot is also used to categorize diseases.

Most of the diseases our European ancestors faced were contagious or infectious, with the worst being the Black Death, the plague that swept through Europe in AD 1348. During these times herbalists were much in demand and they used medicinal and aromatic herbs to cleanse the premises of the sick. For protection, people used herbal oils to fumigate homes but sadly, herbal treatment alone was not enough to save the infected, and thousands died.

Plagues were not the only problem in medieval times; our ancestors used herbs to treat wounds of all kinds, especially battlefield wounds. These were violent times and for serious injuries herb doctors used plants with antiseptic properties such as garlic, lavender, or lemon balm. Cleansing astringents were employed, and a popular one was yarrow, which is a simple meadow herb that was used to treat flesh wounds. An old country name, *soldier's woundwort*, was another name for yarrow, because of its ability to staunch hemorrhages and its power to promote rapid scar tissue healing. The word *anti-septic* speaks for itself; it means "against" sepsis, which causes tissue destruction through bacterial putrefaction. Sepsis can be fatal.

During the First World War, women cultivated healing plants in their gardens and picked herbs to help the wounded when medical supplies were in short supply. Doctors treating the wounded resorted to traditional herbalism when these herbs-of-war were said to have saved lives, and even medical doctors turned to herbs whenever conventional medical supplies ran out. In field hospitals during the tragedy of the Great War, lavender oil was used as a surgical antiseptic.

Soldiers injured in the trenches lost a lot of blood, so the humble stinging nettle was used because of its rich iron content for help during massive blood loss, and also for its diuretic and detoxifying properties. During the war, surgeons who had to operate on wounded soldiers without standard antiseptics used garlic juice on swabs of sphagnum moss in order to prevent sepsis setting in. Garlic was also used during the Second World War to disinfect wounds and prevent gangrene.

In France, until the end of the 19th century, sprigs of rosemary were burned for their purifying properties; the warm, resinous smell, which is similar to incense and honey, could be detected wafting through hospital wards while disinfecting the air. This tradition goes back hundreds of years.

In the 1920s, the famous herbalist, Mrs. Hilda Leyel, opened Culpeper's in Baker Street, London, and she founded the "Society of Herbalists" in 1926 at Culpeper House. Culpeper house was named for Nicholas Culpeper, the famous Elizabethan-era herbalist who is the author of *Culpeper's Complete Herbal*, a classic still in print today, in use for over 360 years. Dame Barbara Cartland, the doyenne of natural health, studied herbal medicine with Mr. Leyel. Dame Barbara lived to be 99 years old and she attributed her good health and longevity to natural medicine. The concept of using plants for healing and the maintenance of vitality was accepted in the United Kingdom before the advent of the National Health Service, and Mrs. Leyel's many herbal books have become standard reference works for herbalists today.

The biochemistry of many plants is still imperfectly understood. For example, the use of the whole plant appears to have stronger healing powers than the extraction and purification of a single ingredient, perhaps because the whole plant's ingredients appear to work more effectively together on a synergistic level.

Modern traditional herbalists believe in the Hippocratic notion of energy and balance. Herbs play a vital role in promoting harmony and well-being of body, mind and spirit, preventing illness, and enhancing health. To an herbalist, healing is a whole body issue that cannot take place unless every body system is in equilibrium. This can only be achieved via a balanced lifestyle that avoids extremes of hot and cold, destructive emotions, poor food choices, and stress.

Herbs Plain and Simple is organized by body system so that you may look up your ailment or area of concern, and read about the recommended herbs for specific conditions. You will find that many of the same herbs pop up in multiple parts of this book, for their beneficial qualities are wide-ranging.

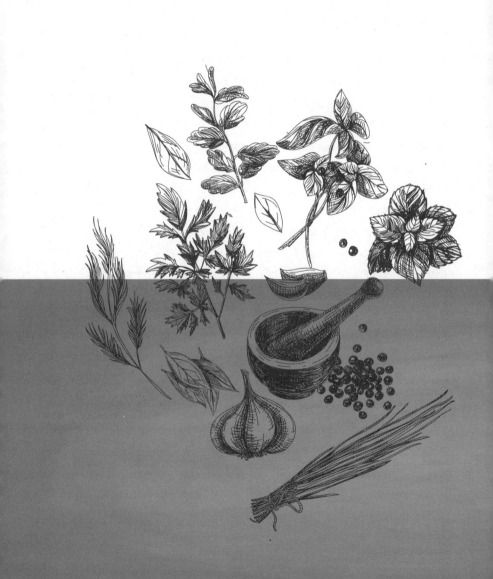

Herbal Healing

2

"Only nature heals."
—School of Hippocrates

In an herbalist's *Materia Medica*, there are many versatile herbs. Some are strengthening restoratives for when we are feeling low, and when we have lost our nerve force there are healing *nervines*. If we are suffering from a blood deficiency, there are herbs that enrich impoverished blood. Some herbs have energy opening abilities, and are able to break up stagnant conditions to get energy flowing again, others have cooling abilities and can be used in hot conditions such as chest colds. Herbs cleanse, nourish, and help the body by tackling the cause of disease. They are created from the sun's energy and are related to nature's cycles. When used for health maintenance they encourage the body's own natural healing processes to restore a healthy balance.

Greek people have always valued herbs as medicines, and today in the remoter villages of the Greek islands markets can

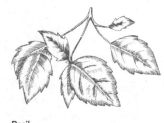

Basil

be found where ancient herbal traditions are still observed. Country peasant women with weather beaten faces are seen selling bunches of freshly picked, fragrant, medicinal herbs gathered from the hillsides. In these markets you will find many herbs, but sweet basil (*Ocimum basilicum*) a most regal herb whose name means "king" in Greek, is especially popular. Used to make delicious St. Basil's bread, the flower tops and leaves of this herb are used medicinally in the treatment of stomach disorders due to basil's antiseptic and sedative properties.

Wild Marjoram (*Origanum vulgare*) is another popular Greek herb. The rose-purple flowers of this herb can be seen on Greek hill slopes and over mountainous regions all over Greece. This gave it the name "Joy of the Mountains," and with its pungent, balsamic aroma, wild marjoram has anti-viral, anti-bacterial properties and is used medicinally to fight infection.

Rosemary

Rosemary (*Rosmarinus officinalis*), another Greek favorite, is used to make a delicious rosemary honey that is taken at the first sign of a cold during the winter months. Rosemary, an anti-microbial, contains immune boosting properties making it a useful herb to use during the cold season. A teaspoon of this honey a day can also soothe stress-related disorders.

Sage (*Salvia officinalis*) is another valued Greek herb that has been used for centuries by Mediterranean families, and is still served today as a fragrant sage tea in cafes throughout Greece. Medicinally it is used for the treatment of colds and as a gargle to soothe sore throats.

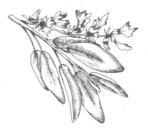

Sage

No Hellenic herb market would be complete without **garlic (*Allium sativum*)**. This much loved botanical; a member of the onion family, and one of the oldest herbs known to humankind, is widely used for culinary and medicinal purposes.

On the island of Ikaria in the North East Aegean, the people are very long-lived. The Ikarians attribute this to a drink made from locally grown medicinal herbs that are brewed into a thick, black, sweet-scented herbal tea. The dried herbs that make up this tea include wildmint, spleenwort, purple sage, rosemary, and a secret ingredient that the people of Ikaria do not divulge. I was told the secret of this longevity tea by my Greek grandmother before she passed away, but I will not reveal it!

Although herbs are nutritive, healing and nourishing to the body, some are poisonous, and I do not advise using any herb picked from the wild or even from a herb garden unless you know what you are doing. The use of the wrong herb could be fatal, so bear this in mind. The herbs that are on display in health shops are safe and they have undergone rigorous and extensive testing.

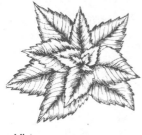

Tablets, liquids, tinctures and herbs packaged in tea bag form are easily available although some are now only available from a qualified herbalist. In my experience tinctures absorb faster than other forms but it is up to you which preparation you choose.

Mint

Popular herbs such as **mint**, **thyme**, **sage,** and **marjoram** are sold for culinary purposes in supermarkets and plant nurseries. These herbs are easy to grow in an herb garden or on a kitchen windowsill. Fresh herbs grown holistically are the most potent. Look for good quality plants when choosing herbs.

By using the entire plant as a medicine, viruses and bacteria find it difficult to develop a way of getting around its therapeutic

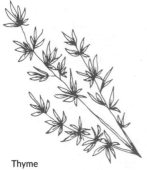

properties, due to the fact that with every harvest there is never quite the same active mix in the plant. It could be because the weather was too wet or too hot, or if it was a good season, then the active principles will be more powerful. In this way, use of the whole plant actually confuses bacteria and viruses. Viruses and bacteria have an innate intelligence that know how

Thyme

to circumvent the compound in a standardized extract, because the composition is always the same. Superbugs have been clever enough to outwit drugs which are standardized. They know what to expect. These organisms have a strong survival mechanism and have mutated in a way that many antibiotics are now no longer a threat to them. This is danger-ous for the human race, as we could go back to a time when alarming infectious diseases that we thought we had conquered return in untreatable form. Using the synergy of the whole plant makes it difficult for bacteria and viruses to develop ways of outmaneuvering and outsmarting the medicinal preparation used to combat disease. Synergistically, their thera-

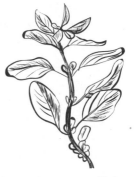

Marjoram

peutic properties enhance one another in a way that their united efforts against disease is greater than they would otherwise be if only one compound of the plant was used alone.

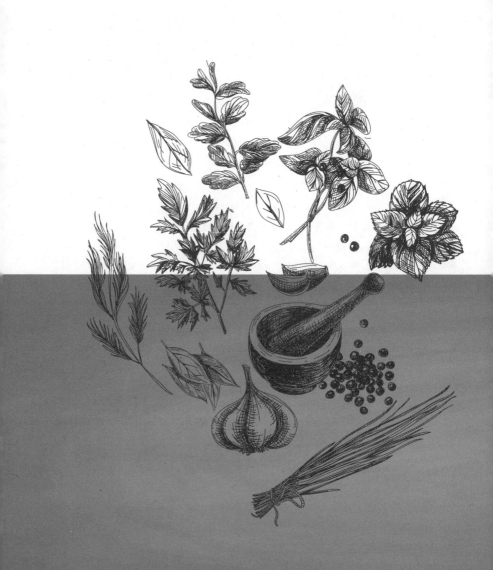

Active Properties of Herbs

3

"All Nature is like one apothecary's shop
covered only with the roof of Heaven"
—Paracelsus

To understand an herb's vital energies and healing potential, some knowledge of the different qualities of each herb is useful. Knowing a little *phytotherapy* from the Greek words for plant, "phyto," and care, "therapy," is valuable for general home use. The potent phyto-chemicals found in plants are divided into groups that indicate an herb's qualities. Herbs are classified as alternatives, bitters, flavonoids, mucilages, saponins, phytosterols, and volatile oils and so on. A number of compounds are used in most herbal medicines as two or more elements tend to produce a greater effect, because by using the whole herb, we draw on its synergistic harmony.

Herbs should be grown in a holistic way, where plants work in harmony with animals, mineral and human kingdoms, in tune with the natural rhythms of the moon, planets and stars. These solar bodies influence the best times to sow, cultivate and harvest herbs.

Herbalists who were in tune with natural rhythms observed that the lunar cycle influenced the life processes of plants. It was noticed that there were times when plant sap was high and at other times low. Traditionally it was thought the sap rose up into plants at full moon and at the new moon the water content of the plant was minimal. Harvesting also took place during the right lunar cycle, and this is still done today in biodynamic farming, which was developed by the Austrian philosopher Rudolf Steiner. Plants and herbs vary with seasonality, weather, growing conditions and other factors. The effectiveness of the plants and herbs differs from year to year. According to Nish Joshi, "biodynamic farming is the oldest non-chemical agricultural movement"

Below are listed some active principles found in health-giving plants. Herbal remedies rely on small quantities of these healing substances for their pharmacological actions. The list gives a brief outline that will help you recognize the group to which a plant belongs and it will assist in identifying its therapeutic principles. The following descriptions show the action and intrinsic character of a, herb.

A Glossary Herbal Properties

This glossary explains herbal properties based on herbalists' knowledge over centuries of use and describes the various actions herbs exert.

Adaptogenic

Adaptogenics increase resilience and resistance against stress, supporting the adrenaline producing glands situated above each kidney, helping the body cope with stress more effectively. They exert an overall normalizing effect, and contribute to body balance, neither over-stimulating nor inhibiting normal body functions.

Alternative

These are blood cleansers, eliminating waste and impurities from blood and lymphatic fluids. Detoxifying, renewing body tissues, alternatives treat toxic conditions. Some stimulate and tone, some relax and purify. Traditional herbalists decide what organ requires elimination of toxic wastes before prescribing the right herb. Alternatives work in conjunction with a healthy diet, stress reduction, and clean air and water.

Note: *Anti* means having the opposite effect, thus against, relieving, or reducing an action.

Anti-catarrhal

Eliminate and reduce the formation and production of mucus, helping expel excess phlegm from the sinuses, lungs, and digestive system. Protecting mucous membranes, anti-catarrhal herbs are often aromatic and astringent in nature.

Anti-microbial

Destroy or inhibit disease-causing micro-organisms helping the body fight off harmful viruses and bacteria. As their name suggests, anti-microbials destroy microbes that cause infectious diseases.

Anti-spasmodic

Prevent or relax spasms, muscle tension, cramp and mild pain within the body.

Anthelmintic

Destroys and expels worms and parasites. These intestinal invaders are still around, especially in the tropics in forms such as bilharzia among others.

Aromatic

Aromatics have a strong, pleasant smell, and a warm, stimulating action, and their agreeable taste and aroma is due to their essential oil content. All have antiseptic and antimicrobial properties helping the immune system by increasing white blood cell production. Circulation boosters, stimulating expectoration, they help improve appetite, digestion, and absorption.

Anti-rheumatic

Relieve rheumatism and arthritis, working in a gentler way than anti-inflammatories and steroids.

Astringent

Astringents, due to their drying effect, contract tissue, thus reducing discharges. They offer protection and healing via their binding action on inflamed mucous membranes and arrest bleeding.

Note: Serious and unstoppable bleeding requires attention from a qualified medical practitioner.

Bitters

These aid digestion and liver function. Cooling in nature, they encourage secretion of digestive juices. Bitters help bile flow to the liver and are sedative and relaxant, or anti-inflammatory. Cooling herbs slow down body processes and soothe irritation.

Carminative

Carminatives ease spasm and tension in the digestive tract, thus reducing flatulence. Their volatile oils affect the digestive system by toning mucous membranes and increasing peristalsis, the muscular activity of the gut that propels waste content onward.

Demulcent

Demulcents soothe and protect dry irritated tissues and mucous membranes. They have a moisturizing action.

Diaphoretics

Internal cleansers, diaphoretics induce sweating by eliminating toxic wastes via the pores of the skin and kidneys. Widely used in feverish conditions, they reduce a high temperature and help the circulation regain equilibrium.

Diuretic

Diuretics promote the flow of urine; they reduce puffiness caused by retention of fluid in body tissues.

Emmenagogue

These herbs promote menstrual flow, and work by stimulating and eliminating congested endometrium (the lining of the uterus). Helpful in pelvic congestion and period pains. They are contraindicated in pregnancy.

Expectorant

Promote expulsion of mucus and difficult to remove sticky phlegm from the lungs and throat.

Febrifuge

Helpful in reducing fevers, these herbs are useful during infections.

Flavonoids

Flavonoids are the colored pigments present in fruits and vegetables. When Grandma said "put color on your plate" she was right! Wide ranging in effect, they benefit the heart and circulatory system, lowering blood pressure, strengthening capillary fragility and blood vessel walls. Many flavonoid rich plants are diuretic, antispasmodic, and anti-inflammatory.

Galactogogue

Increase breast milk flow in nursing mothers. Taken as tinctures or teas.

Hepatic

Hepatic herbs tone and strengthen liver function and promote bile flow (a greenish-yellow alkaline fluid secreted by the liver cells).

Hypotensive

Help lower high blood pressure.

Immune-System Stimulants

Strengthening in action, these herbs help fight off invading infections. They have immune boosting powers.

Lymphatics

These herbs exert their influence on the lymphatic system, clearing swollen lymph nodes, particularly after infections.

Mucilages

Their gel-like substance soothes, relaxes, and protects mucous membranes. They increase fluids in dried out membranes and have a cooling effect. Their sticky, viscous sap calms inflamed surfaces and exert a palliative effect on the digestive, respiratory, and urinary systems.

Nervines

Nervines and herbal nerve tonics support nervous system function, and by calming nerves, they benefit stress-related conditions and are useful relaxants or sedatives, easing nervous tension, excitability, and inducing sleep. They also act as stimulants, so due to their complex properties nervine herbs can bring an imbalanced system back into harmony, restoring emotional stability if nerves need calming or adding vitality if energies are depleted. Nervines are useful for nerve repair (see chapter 12, The Nervous System).

Nutritive

Nourishing in action, the nurturing and sustaining properties of these herbs provide the body with nourishment and stimulate metabolic processes.

Tonic

Invigorating, restoring, strengthening, tonics reinstate energy to a depleted system. They promote the workings of body systems, improving the function of a specific organ, nourishing overall vigor, and boosting strength and well-being. They can be used as a pick-me-up when the system is in need of energizing. Tonic herbs have a strong cleansing action.

Saponins

From the Latin *sapo* meaning "soap." Saponins produce a soap-like frothing lather when mixed with water. Softening, cleansing, expectorants, saponin rich herbs increase bronchial secretions, expelling sticky mucus and normalizing glands.

Sedative

These herbs quiet the nervous system with their calming and relaxing effect. They subdue restlessness, excitability, hyperactivity, and help induce restful sleep.

Stimulant

Any substance that increases activity, body strength, and energy is known as a stimulant. These herbs help spur a sluggish circulatory system and increase energy.

Tannins

Sour tasting astringent substances, tannins bind with proteins on the skin and mucous membranes forming a protective layer. Their astringency contracts body tissues, thus creating resistance to microbial invasion and deterring fluid secretions.

Vulnerary

These herbs encourage wound healing and promote cell growth and repair.

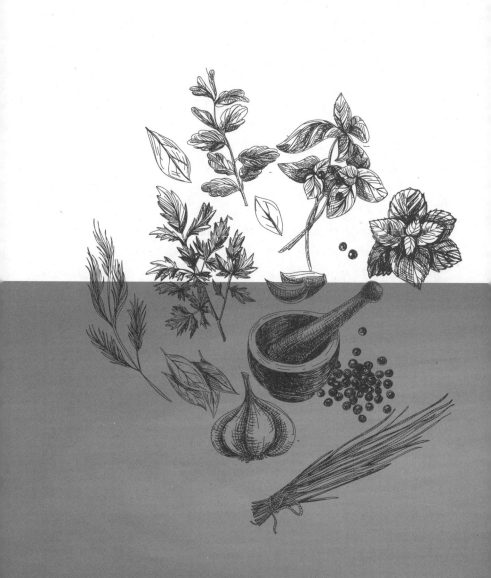

A
Green
Pharmacy

4

"Look deep into nature, then you will
understand everything better."
—Albert Einstein

Growing herbs in the garden is a therapeutic pleasure and an opportunity to relax and feel at one with nature's rhythms. Herbs are not difficult to grow. Culinary herbs to add zest to your cooking, while those you grow for medicinal use will help you create your own green garden pharmacy. Herbs can also be grown for their sheer beauty, scent, and ornamental value. Just the sight and heady scent of a beautiful variety of plants growing in your garden can lift your spirits.

An interesting piece of folklore tells us that herb gardens were designed in narrow beds that were crisscrossed with paths. Two paths often intersected to form a cross, because it was believed that this would scare the devil away.

Healing plants can be grown successfully in a window box, and growing your own herbs assures you of their freshness and potency. You can start with some easily available culinary herbs, such as parsley, rosemary, sage, and thyme. You will find these in any supermarket, garden center, or herb nursery. Easy to grow in pots or on a warm windowsill, they can be used in cooking or for herbal teas. For infusions (herbal teas) chop freshly picked herbs and add them to boiling water. Small teapots with built-in-strainers are ideal. Dried herbs can also be used. Dried medicinal herbs can also be bought from specialist herb suppliers.

If feeling in a creative mood you can design a theme for your herb garden. You can choose aromatic plants that have a strong fragrance such as chamomile, lavender, or lemon balm. You can design a bee garden, with bee-friendly plants that will help ensure the survival of these endangered creatures. Planting bee-friendly herbs in your garden will encourage these important pollinators to make a bee-line to your garden. Bees love lemon balm, with its musky lemon scent. Other herbs like rosemary, borage, thyme, marjoram, and mint will also attract bees to your garden. Or you could design a garden based on medieval herb gardens where apothecaries grew dandelion, yarrow, nettles, and other medicinal herbs. Even if your garden is small or has poor soil this should not be a problem as most herbs are hardy. Many grow well in pots or containers, including parsley, peppermint, oregano, basil, feverfew, and lemon verbena.

The medicinal value of an herb is affected by the weather, the cycles of the moon, and the seasons of the year. With experience, you will gain invaluable knowledge of how to grow and gather plants for home use.

Herbal preparations can be made into healing infusions, tinctures, decoctions (also called elixirs), and poultices. Identification of each herb along with knowledge of when and how best to collect it is important when considering using herbs for therapeutic purposes. Herbs such as thyme, hyssop, tarragon, mint, marjoram, and basil are easy to grow. Another easy-to-grow plant is chamomile, which is popularly made into an herbal tea. It is a low-growing herb with a fine feathery appearance, and it releases a pleasant apple scent if squeezed. In the past, village wise women called chamomile "the plant physician" because they noticed its healing effect extending to ailing plants growing next to it.

Chamomile

Herbs should be harvested just before the buds open into full flower. This maintains the essential oils and retains the full flavor.

Delivery Methods

There is an assortment of delivery methods that have been developed by herbalists, and I have listed some of them below.

Extract

A concentrated form of an herb that is obtained by mixing the herb with alcohol and/or water. Usually made from stimulating or antispasmodic herbs.

Decoction (elixir)

Suitable for hard plant materials, such as berries, roots, barks, seeds, all of which require longer extraction to access their healing action. Cover the chopped herb with boiling water, simmer gently for twenty to thirty minutes, and then strain.

Infusion

Standard tea preparation suitable for fresh or dried leaves, flowers, aerial parts (above ground), and fine roots. Infusions are a simple way of preparing tea. Pour boiling water over finely chopped herbs, cover with a lid and leave to infuse for a few minutes.

Ointment

Powdered plant parts added to an oily substance and applied topically.

Poultice

Fresh or dried plants are applied to the skin warm or hot in order to improve local circulation, ease pain and inflammation, draw out toxins or foreign bodies, heal bruising, swelling and wounds. Made with damp plant material, which has been strained out of an infusion/decoction.

Powder

Dried herbs traditionally pulverized in a mortar and pestle.

Syrup

Plant parts added to honey or a sugar water mixture.

Tincture

Herbs dissolved in brandy, wine, vodka, or vinegar are called tinctures. The healing property of the herb is extracted and preserved in your chosen medium. They remain potent for many years and tinctures made this way have an advantage over a water-based preparation.

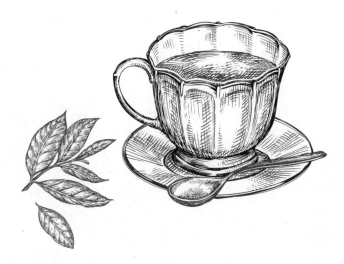

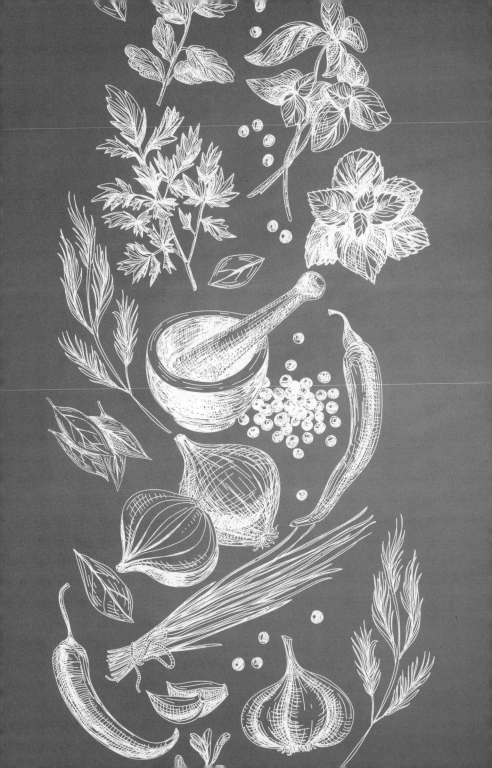

Part Two

HERBS FOR DIFFERENT BODY SYSTEMS

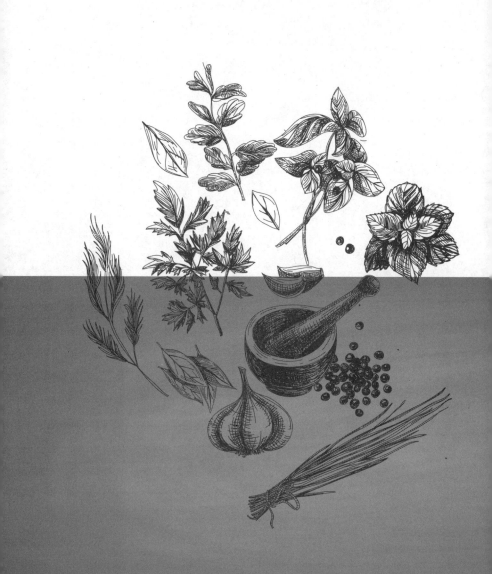

Using Herbs to Heal the Body

5

*"Man can provide medicine & show direction,
but only nature can truly heal."*
—Dr. A. Vogel, Naturopath

In the following chapters, herbs are discussed according to each of the body systems: immune, circulatory, digestive, respiratory, and so forth. Herbalism is an all-inclusive mode of healing that takes into account the whole physical body, as well as emotions, mind, and spirit. This is where this therapy differs from conventional health care. It is a different type of medicine, with a supportive action on the body's recuperative powers. Herbal medicine is concerned with preventing illness as well as curing it, and making use of a wide range of botanic medicines to maintain your body's systems will help you improve your health and stay well.

Seasonal Changes

Herbs can be used for a detox when over-indulgence during the holiday celebrations may have left you feeling a little bloated and lethargic. They are an effective detox during cold and damp weather when a heavier, "comfort food" diet results in accumulated toxins, which need to be eliminated. The liver is key to the body's cleansing system, and a short course of a liver boosting herb such as milk thistle will help support this important organ, helping to relieve symptoms of over- eating and drinking. There are a number of detoxing herbs to bring your health back into balance during the first month of the year, and maintaining a detox routine throughout the year can greatly improve your general well-being and promote good health. Make this one of your New Year resolutions!

When the dark days of winter give way to the life force of spring—a time of new beginnings, growth, and regeneration— cleansing herbs act as spring purifiers that detox a lethargic system and help improve our energy. Spring tonics as a pick-me-up during this season of increasing warmth should include purifying herbs with cleansing properties that help increase vitality, preparing us for the change of seasons to come. This is the time for a real spring clean!

During summer, there are cooling herbs for an overheated system. These herbs are used for slowing down or relaxing the body and cooling down heat (yang energies). Cooling herbs such as sweet basil can be used in salads during this season of the year when people tend to eat more fresh plant foods.

During autumn, herbs to prepare for the coming winter can be used to fortify the body, enabling it to cope with cold and flu bugs that abound during this time of year. If people have prepared themselves with plant remedies for the shorter darker days, they may find they develop fewer colds and avoid seasonal affective disorder (SAD). This is a form of winter depression that brings low mood, sleep problems, and fatigue due to the lack of sun having an have an effect on the brain's biochemistry. Herbs that can alleviate the winter blues and uplift mood are well worth a try.

Every change of season is accompanied by an energy shift, and it is good to know that there are herbs that can help us achieve a fortifying effect on the body, cleansing, building, uplifting our mood, and reinstating harmony. These seasonal cycles are represented not only in the different phases of the year but also the energy alterations our bodies undergo with each seasonal transition. Various different herbs can provide significant support during these changeovers to help keep our body systems working well.

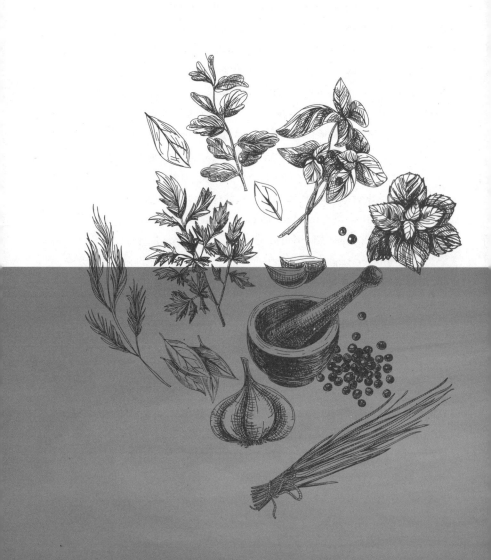

The Immune System

6

"True wisdom consists in not departing from nature."

—Seneca

The key to a robust immune system lies in a healthy lifestyle, wholesome diet, and plenty of exercise with a minimum of stress. This system and its relation to other parts of the body is considered the major player in traditional herbalism. Without a healthy functioning immune system, no other body system can exhibit optimum health.

Traditional herbalists believe in "the three R's"—*resistance, repair, and recovery.* We use herbs to build up our *resistance* if we fall ill, herbs to *repair* body tissues during and after illness, and herbs that assist *recovery* to get us back on track.

The immune system encompasses the entire body, as it includes the lymphatic system and associated organs. Without a strong immune system we would be unable to fight off even simple organisms. Nature provides us with immune stimulants and modulators from the plant world that have been used in folk medicine for a long time. Allergic conditions, such as hay fever or asthma, result when the immune system is not in balance and is overreacting. Reinstating stability through the use of herbs that dampen down this over-active immune response may help to alleviate these unpleasant symptoms.

Immune Enhancing Herbs

A number of herbs have been shown to have immune-boosting powers. They can help prevent colds or significantly reduce the duration of one. These immune enhancing herbs have also been shown to speed up recovery, helping us overcome illness and restoring health and well-being. Here are some winter essentials that will offer support during this seasonal change when infections tend to become more prevalent. These will help you to prepare and strengthen yourself against the cold and flu bugs that spread so quickly during this less than healthy time of year.

Echinacea (Echinacea Purpurea/E. Angustifolia)— Immune System Protector

Echinacea, known also as purple coneflower, was used by Native Americans to treat snakebites and poisonous infections. Colonial settlers recognized echinacea's benefits and appreciated its powerful healing abilities. Today this immune supporting herb is very popular. It is generally known for its anti-bacterial and anti-viral properties, but echinacea is also effective in its ability to act as a lymphatic cleanser. Echinacea stimulates the body's immune system response to flu, colds, and upper respiratory tract infections. Those who are prone to colds and infections would be wise to take a course of echinacea for a couple of weeks at a time to stimulate the immune system. This herb protects mucous membranes and tissue barriers, increasing interferon (a protein released from virus infected cells that interferes with the growth of the virus) activating special immune cells with specific anti-viral, and anti-bacterial chemicals, and helping strengthen immune function.

Feeling lethargic and run down after a bout of flu? Echinacea with its blood detoxifying properties and purifying actions can help restore strength, providing some support for that under-the-weather feeling. Its cleansing abilities sweep away toxic residues after an infection. A course for a number of weeks may be needed to help build up and tone the whole body after a period of ill health. It is available in capsules, liquid extract, teas, and tinctures. Used for upper respiratory tract infections, influenza and colds, this herb can help give symptomatic relief.

Elderberry (Sambucus nigra)—Herb of Elders

The name of the elderberry originates from the word "elder" because it was believed that it promoted longevity. Known as a gypsy remedy for colds and flu, it was made into a traditional formula for coughs and bronchial infections by these resourceful people. Elderberry juice was pressed from the tree's berries, boiled with honey, and made into an herbal syrup cold remedy. Gypsy wisdom passed this formula down through the generations, and today science has isolated two active ingredients from the black elderberry that can stop a virus by preventing it penetrating cell walls. It appears to combat free radicals and inflammation, relieves coughs and congestion and enhances immune system function. It is effective against flu viruses and soothes the respiratory tract, stimulating circulation. Wise gypsy lore has now been proven to be right! Take this good immune booster as a preventative during the winter season. You can take this in the form of tablets, capsules, syrups, and teas.

Garlic (Allium sativum)—Nature's Immunizer

Garlic has been used for thousands of years as both food and medicine. Ancient records show that for over 5,000 years, garlic's healing qualities have been treating disease. Culpeper described garlic as a "remedy for all diseases and hurts but whose heat was very vehement." Strong smelling with a sharp flavor, garlic is not to everyone's taste. This may be why it was called "stinking rose" and used to ward off vampires! Popular in monastic gardens all over medieval Europe, harvested bulbs were used to treat wandering beggars. In monastery kitchens a garlic smell wafted throughout the cloisters, where the smell was thought to prevent infection spreading within the confines of the living quarters. Garlic is particularly helpful with respiratory problems, helping to promote healing and restore health to this delicate area.

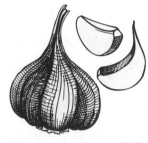

Garlic

Garlic is a complex herb containing numerous warming and therapeutic chemical compounds. In traditional Chinese Medicine, garlic is considered yang (hot) and used in cold, damp conditions. A heating herb, garlic speeds up body processes, increasing circulation and is stimulating in nature. A strong herbal antibiotic, it is used by herbalists for the treatment of colds, flu, respiratory, and circulatory problems. Garlic assists the body's natural protective action, particularly in chesty colds and catarrh, as it not only keeps colds and infections at bay but also helps push them out of the system, helping to speed up recovery. Garlic's compounds, particularly its therapeutic ingredient allicin, which is released when the bulb is crushed, makes this herb an effective medicine. Allicin encourages the white blood cells of the immune system to reproduce, boosting the body's defense system. Modern nutritional science has proven that regular ingestion of garlic can lower levels of "bad" LDL cholesterol.

If your immune system falters and a cold or chill sets in, some garlic will provide a welcome relief to unpleasant symptoms such as catarrh, runny nose, and troublesome coughs. Make use of nature's powerful immunizer as a preventative. Taken regularly, a little garlic a day keeps the doctor away! Tablets, capsules, tinctures, and cough mixtures are available from health stores while fresh cloves can be bought at supermarkets. Combines well with Echinacea.

Ashwagandha Root (Withania somnifera)—Indian Ginseng

In India Ashwagandha, a plant belonging to the nightshade family, is known as Indian ginseng. Growing in tough conditions, this plant has the ability to survive harsh environments and its nourishing properties have been recognized for thousands of years. An adaptogen, the roots and berries are used for medicine. There

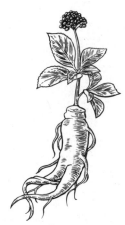

is evidence that Ashwagandha has a sedative, calming effect and also a tonic effect which boosts the immune system. Ginseng improves immunity when this system has been weakened through over work, illness, or just run down. This herb's harmonizing properties are useful for promoting inner strength and stamina.

Ashwagandha belongs to the Ayurvedic pharmacopoeia and is used for its immune boosting power. A course of Ashwaganda would be well worth taking during the winter to help strengthen the body's own powers of resistance. It will help promote vital-

Ashwagandha ginseng

ity, vigor, restful sleep, and mental clarity. The key to successful prevention is a body system in balance and harmony. Take some Ashwagandha, a powerful immune strengthener, when you need some immune support. Available as tablets or purchased from Ayurvedic practitioners as a powdered root to be made into a tea. Note that the fresh ginseng commonly available in supermarkets is Panax ginseng, not Ashwagandha. The more common Panax ginseng is discussed in chapters 20 and 21.

Allergies

Allergic disorders are due to an over-reaction of the immune system. Allergies seem to have become a modern epidemic. Traditional Chinese medicine terms allergies as a hot condition due to swelling, over activity, and burning, which means that allergies require cooling herbs. Using immune modulators has shown that they are particularly useful when the immune system has been weakened and its protective abilities lessened through stress, poor diet, or other lifestyle factors.

Hay fever (or seasonal rhinitis) with sneezing, itchy eyes, runny nose, wheezing, and frequent infections, are all symptoms of a weakened immune system or an over-reactive one. There is a wide selection of time-tested herbs to choose from for infection treatment or prevention, as well as herbal modulators that act by helping to dampen down an over-reactive immune system. A teaspoon of a good quality, local, raw unprocessed honey taken before and during the hay fever season has been found to help some people.

Eyebright (Euphrasia officinalis)—Herb of Gladness

Euphrasia or eyebright is an herb whose name is derived from the Greek *euphrosyne*, meaning "gladness." This herb grows in meadows and grasslands in the United States and Britain. This herb's flower, with yellow and purple markings and a black center, had a bloodshot look and resembles a human eye. According to the *Doctrine of Signatures*, eyebright—"the gladdener"—was used to treat eye ailments and used as an eye tonic.

Eyebright's astringent properties are ideal for relieving excess mucus associated with allergic sinusitis. In hay fever, when eyes are inflamed, itchy, streaming, and sore, soothing eyebright eye drops can be beneficial. Each summer, allergy sufferers routinely take eyebright to help control allergic symptoms. A qualified herbalist can make up an eyebright lotion or eye drops.

Nettle (Urtica dioica)—Allergy Buster

Stinging nettles, which we consider common weeds, have many medicinal actions. The value of nettles was well known throughout history, and Samuel Pepys wrote in his diary in 1661 that he enjoyed "nettle porridge." I am not sure whether we would enjoy

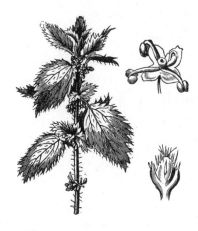

Nettle

this today! Acting as restorative tonics and natural diuretics, nettles are rich in iron. Nettles are helpful is alleviating allergic reactions. Allergies are problems that affect many people during spring and summer, particularly if they live in areas where they are likely to come into contact with excess pollen. Allergic symptoms are distressing, with acute catarrhal congestion, runny nose and eyes, and sneezing, all of which cause misery and discomfort.

Before spring begins, building up resistance with a course of anti-allergy herbs may help prevent the onset of hay fever or avert the sting of a more severe attack. Nettle is known for its-antihistamine action and it helps reduce sensitivity to pollens because of its marked anti-allergenic action. This herb is an excellent example of a normalizer, an herbal remedy that supports health and helps maintain the immune system's balance. This herbal tonic food nourishes the body with its immune-strengthening actions due to its iron, calcium and silica content. Nettle is available in the form of tablets, tinctures, and tea.

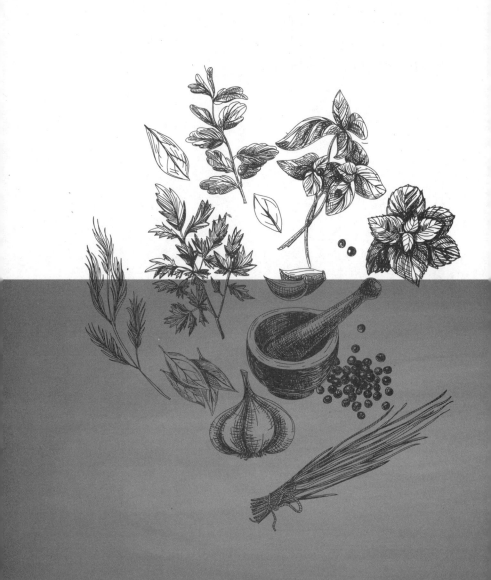

The Heart and Circulatory System

7

*"Nature, time, and patience are
the three greatest physicians."*
—Irish Proverb

The heart and circulatory system are concerned with carrying various nutrients and oxygen to and from different parts of the body via the bloodstream, and this vital transport system also removes waste product from every cell. It is important that we look after the heart and circulation with a wholesome diet and the use of appropriate herbal remedies that have an affinity with this system. Common conditions that affect circulation are chilblains, poor blood flow to the hands and feet, blood pressure, high cholesterol levels, and varicose veins. Many people suffer from poor circulation, and looking after our cardiovascular system should be a health priority.

The lymphatic system is intimately connected with the circulatory system, but unlike blood circulation it does not have a pump (a heart), so slow-moving lymph fluid needs to be kept in motion in order to remove cellular debris if the body is to stay healthy. Exercise and massage are recommended to keep lymphatic structures moving, and we will discuss this further in chapter 10.

The Three G's for Healthy Circulation

Garlic (Allium sativum)—Heart Protector

I have already mentioned garlic's immune supporting benefits. Allicin is one of the most powerful active principals of garlic. It protects the heart, and this versatile herb's other therapeutic property ajoene, which is also a heart protector. Allicin, as it breaks down its by-products, is believed to interact with a body chemical that regulates blood clotting, helping to keep this mechanism balanced. Garlic protects blood vessels, keeping them

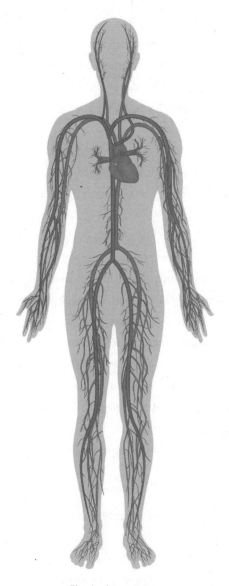

The circulatory system

healthy into old age, and it also has cholesterol lowering abilities, making it a valuable aid to keeping the heart healthy. Due to its artery-dilating properties, garlic can also help lower blood pressure. Researchers discovered that eating garlic is cardio-protective, something herbalists have known since the early part of the 20th century.

When we ingest garlic, allicin breaks down into sulphur compounds, which react with red blood cells and produce hydrogen sulphide. This relaxes blood vessels, keeping blood flowing easily. Research on garlic was carried out by the University of Alabama, Birmingham, and it appeared in *Proceedings of the National Academy of Sciences*; meanwhile as far back as 1982, *The British Medical Journal* endorsed garlic's properties in lowering cholesterol and reducing blood pressure by dilating blood vessels.

Garlic has so many benefits that go a long way to helping avoid heart attacks and strokes, and it would be wise to take some garlic as a preventative on a regular basis. The primary goal of herbalism is to strengthen the person's own bodily functions before disease sets in; using herbs is a prophylactic (a preventative).

Fresh garlic cloves are available from supermarkets, and tablets, capsules, and tinctures are available in health stores.

Ginger (Zingiber officinalis)—Eastern Spice

This herb with its warming qualities is one of nature's most valued plants. Used in Chinese and Ayurvedic medicine for thousands of years, we find its use in records dating from the 4th century BC. Ginger's fiery, stimulating properties can help bring warmth to the whole body, stimulating sluggish blood circulation, and supporting healthy heart function. Ginger warms up peripheral circulation, improving cold hands and feet, and is good to use if you suffer from chilblains. This aromatic spice also helps support the maintenance of healthy blood pressure and cholesterol levels. This finding is supported by a study published in the *New England Journal of Medicine*, which found that ginger helps reduce cholesterol. It can also help lower blood pressure and prevent blood clots that trigger heart attacks and strokes.

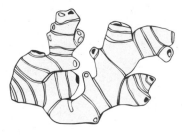

Ginger root

Ginger adds zest to herbal teas and taken with some honey can help stave off winter chills. Traditional Chinese herbalists use this yang herb to stimulate sweating through the skin and to stimulate the heart. They also recommend a course of ginger throughout the winter to warm up body energies during the cold and damp season. You can make infusions from fresh root, or buy capsules, tinctures, and ginger tea.

Ginkgo Biloba—Mankind's Sacred Tree

One of the world's oldest living species of tree, ginkgo biloba has spread its protective branches over the earth for three thousand years. It was believed that this sacred tree of Asia protected Japanese and Chinese temples from evil spirits, while gingko's health-related properties were recognized by ancient Traditional Chinese herbalists. The roots and bark contain beneficial flavonoids.

In the West, ginkgo has become popular and is used to improve circulation to all parts of the body. Because of its blood-moving abilities, it is beneficial for use by people who suffer from cold hands and feet. Ginkgo strengthens and opens up blood vessels. Traditional herbalists recommend ginkgo to help move stagnant

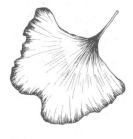

Ginkgo

energy. After a heart attack, ginkgo helps repair damaged blood vessels and tissues. Ginkgo can be taken as a brain food to improve blood flow to the brain, helping to boost concentration and to slow dementia that comes with old age. It also has a positive effect on mental performance, and it protects aging brains by supporting brain function and improving memory. Problems with tinnitus, an inner ear condition that can sometimes also be age-related, has also been helped with the use of this herb. Extracts of ginkgo biloba are available as tinctures, capsules, tablets and teas.

Other Beneficial Herbs

Cayenne (Capsicum annum)—Blood Mover

Capsicum, commonly known as cayenne pepper, was used by ancient herbalists to treat the "King's evil" or scrofula. This small perennial shrub originated from the tropical areas of South America, and today this kitchen spice is used to flavor food— for those who can stand the heat! It was the great standby of traditional herbalists, who used it when dealing with cholera. Medicinally, this warming herb promotes a healthy circulatory system due to its active properties, imparting warmth to a number of body functions. Exerting a beneficial effect on the cardiovascular system, it invigorates the blood and helps remove toxins, substances that undermine health. Cayenne improves circulation, and helps open up body tissues, improving blood flow, which is why traditional herbalists consider cayenne a good blood mover. Cayenne acts as a catalyst, breaking down food and aiding its absorption; it also improves lung resistance against cold and damp. A good circulatory tonic to use when this system needs a boost. It is available in capsules or tinctures from health stores. Capsicum combines well with garlic.

Hawthorn (Crataegus oxyacantha)—May Blossom Tree

Hawthorn is a common hedgerow shrub that is known as the May blossom tree. In Pagan traditions, hawthorn was used in fertility rites and was a symbol of both life and death. The hawthorn tree flowered on May Day and was used to decorate the maypole.

This warming herb's red haw berries contain valuable flavonoids and tannins that are attributed to improving peripheral circulation, regulating the heart rate and blood pressure. Rich in vitamins C and B-complex, hawthorn has diuretic properties and is good for minor angina (although hawthorn should *never* replace a prescription for nitro-glycerin tablets). The main medicinal properties of this plant are its tonic flavonoids, which help prevent coronary artery disease. This wayside herb has been used by traditional herbalists as a restorative and strengthener for various heart problems. Hawthorn normalizes and strengthens the contractions of the cardiac muscle, and it is a valued natural medicine used as a heart tonic due to its invigorating action on this vital organ. It is available as a tea, in tablets, capsules, or as tinctures.

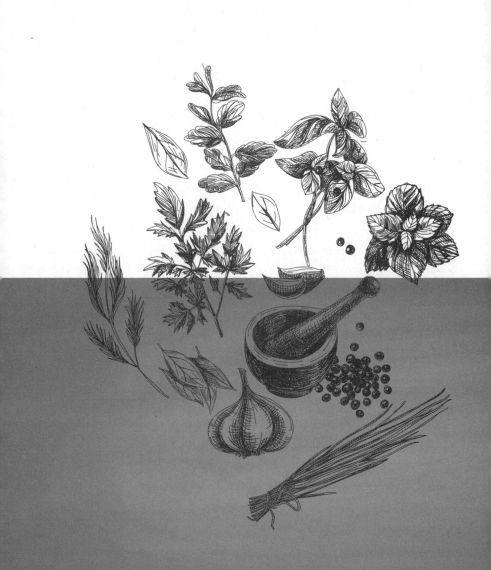

The Digestive System

8

"Everything in excess is opposed by Nature."
—Hippocrates

The digestive system is dedicated to breaking down food and allowing its nutrients to be absorbed into the bloodstream, from where they are then carried to every part of the body. This system is subject to a variety of problems and it is important that it is functioning well for the health of the whole body.

Stomach pain due to ulcers and indigestion from over eating, irritable bowel syndrome (IBS), constipation, and diarrhea are just some of the problems that can plague this sensitive area. The liver, which is part of digestion, gets special attention in this chapter. The liver is an amazing chemical factory performing more than five hundred major tasks, using thousands of different enzymes. The liver plays a vital role as a filtering system for the blood.

There are a number of herbs that can help improve the function of the digestive system, and each has a unique purpose in digestive health and detoxification support.

Artichoke (Cynara scolymus)—Nature's Liver Tonic

Legend has it that the mighty god Zeus was rejected by the object of his desire, the beautiful Cynara, so he turned her into a thistle and thus created the artichoke plant!

The artichoke has been used medicinally since the time of the Roman Empire. Belonging to the daisy family, artichoke can grow up to six feet high. The medicinal qualities of this plant are well recognized, and the first mention of artichoke's health benefits was documented by pupils of the Greek philosopher Aristotle.

Used as a liver tonic, artichoke's restorative power improves liver health. It stimulates bile flow, thus leading to better digestion and helping the body break down food and alcohol more effectively. This herb also strengthens liver and kidney function.

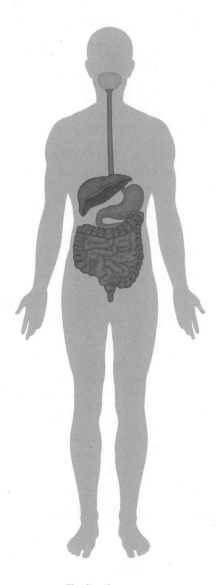

The digestive system

Artichoke's active properties have many benefits, but its main ingredient is cynarin. High concentrations of cynarin are found in the leaves, and they can be used to improve appetite and digestion. Their bitterness has a stimulating effect on the liver and also a cooling action. Artichoke appears to be helpful in alleviating symptoms of irritable bowel syndrome, improving nausea, bloating, constipation, and pain from gas. Research has shown that, taken to help maintain a healthy digestive system, artichoke may also help maintain cholesterol at normal levels. Artichoke extracts are available in tablets and tinctures from health stores.

Dandelion (Taraxacum officinalis)—Lion's Tooth

The name of this flower is derived from the French "*dent de lion*" meaning lion's tooth. This name was supposedly given to this plant by a 15th century surgeon, due to the dandelion's jagged shaped leaves. Folk healers have long prescribed the root of this cleansing herb for liver and digestive problems.

Today this herb is used for its diuretic properties, which have now been confirmed scientifically. Dandelion restores potassium rather than depleting it like conventional diuretics do, and it promotes healthy digestive functioning. A large part of the immune system is connected to the digestive system, and both are intricately woven, so if one is imbalanced the other is affected.

Dandelion coffee made from the roasted roots is a renowned liver tonic and detoxifier. Dandelion tea made from dried leaves and taken regularly throughout the day helps the body excrete excess fluids through urination.

This herb is also useful for premenstrual bloating caused by an excess of fluid build-up prior to a menstrual period. Dandelion is available in the form of tea or as tablets, tinctures, and dandelion root coffee from health stores. It combines well with nettle, working together to purify the blood.

Ginger (Zingiber officinale)—Warming Yang Herb

We have already met this amazing warming spice under the section on the circulatory system. This root was introduced into Europe during the Roman Empire, and it has held an honored place in traditional medicine for digestive problems for a very long time. Chinese herbalists have used ginger root for 2,000 years, and the ancient Greeks prized it as an aid to digestion, mixing powdered ginger into bread.

Growing wild in Asia, ginger's unique properties and therapeutic benefits are now being rediscovered and confirmed scientifically. Today it is used therapeutically to alleviate nausea and upset stomach, due to its anti-emetic properties, and it is also used to alleviate stomach cramps. Gingerols and zingerones are the active anti-inflammatory constituents of this pungent spice. It is a natural remedy for heartburn, as well as nausea caused by motion sickness, so it is helpful for travelers. As a digestive tonic, ginger helps normalize the digestive process. Before eating anything, the wise sage Confucius would ginger up his food by sprinkling a little of this yang spice onto his meal. He knew that some ginger would promote appetite, prevent nausea, and help expel gases from the stomach and intestinal tract.

Ginger root can be bought in any supermarket. The root can be grated and made into a warming ginger tea that is helpful for soothing nausea.

Slippery Elm Bark (Ulmus fulva)—Gut Soother

Native Americans used the powdered inner bark of the elm tree to make poultices to soothe damaged skin and to draw out poisons from boils and abscesses. European settlers used it to calm the terrible digestive problems of typhoid sufferers. Today this herb is a popular remedy for digestive discomfort, such as acid dyspepsia, irritable bowel syndrome, or for the type of problems associated with eating a food that disagrees with you.

Soothing, nutritive, and demulcent in action, slippery elm bark has calming properties. Its moisturizing action eases an upset digestion, protects the stomach and eases diarrhea and intestinal cramps. It neutralizes acidity, coating the mucous membrane lining of the gastrointestinal tract. A gentle form of non-digestible carbohydrate, it makes its way through the gut, flushing out toxic wastes as it transits through the digestive system.

Slippery elm also works as an expectorant by increasing bronchial secretions, loosening up thick and stubborn throat mucus, decreasing the stickiness of troublesome phlegm, and helping the body to remove it.

Slippery elm bark comes in powder form and it can be used to make a soothing tea for irritation of the digestive tract. The powder can be sprinkled on muesli or oatmeal, helpful in healing the lining of the gut in leaky gut syndrome.

Milk Thistle (Silybum marianum)—Liver Reviver

This herb is a flowering plant of the daisy family, and it has been used for hundreds of years as a liver strengthener and to treat various liver disorders due to its significant liver-protective actions.

Strange powers were attributed to the milk thistle in medieval times, possibly because it was found growing in graveyards and cloister gardens.

The liver has to work hard to detoxify the body, and this herb's active property, a flavonoid known as silymarin, has been shown to maintain the health of liver cells and to neutralize the effect of toxins. It has a digestive "bitter tonic" action, helping promote the flow of bile in liver disorders. A popular herbal remedy today, it is used to help maintain a healthy liver and for the relief of an upset stomach or indigestion.

Peppermint (Mentha piperita)—Digestive tonic

The Greek doctor, Dioscorides, is reputed to have regularly worn a sprig of peppermint to lift his spirits. Its antispasmodic actions were recognized by physicians of the ancient world, and peppermint was popular with our more modern ancestors who saw it as a healing herb for the relief of digestive colic, sluggish digestion, flatulence, and bloating. Used for centuries as a gastrointestinal aid, peppermint helps relax the muscles of the digestive tract and stimulates bile flow.

Today this herb is sold to relieve indigestion, soothe stomach-ache, and relieve colicky diarrhea. Studied extensively, peppermint oil has been accepted as a treatment for irritable bowel syndrome, as the volatile oils help to ease bloating, cramps, and spasms.

Peppermint can be taken in hot infusions (dried herb in boiling water) or used to make a peppermint tea (using commercially made tea bags). It is usually available as enteric coated capsules for the relief of IBS, available in health stores.

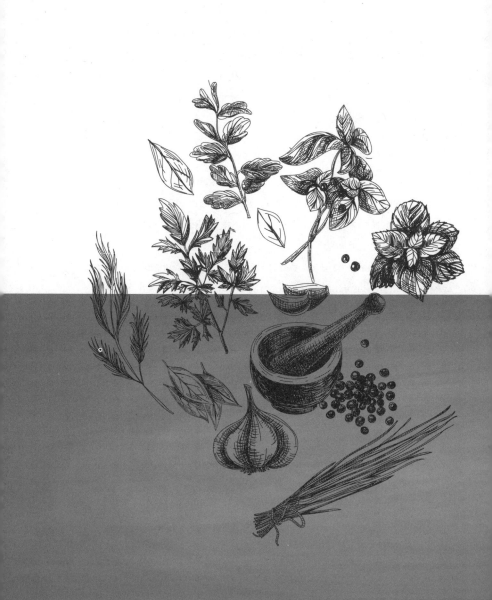

The Endocrine System

9

"The first wealth is health."
—Ralph Waldo Emerson

The endocrine system resides in the brain, chest, abdominal, and pelvic cavities and it consists of a series of separate but related hormone secreting glands. These glands control many of the body's systems, helping to keep all body structures working well. The main function of the glandular system is to produce chemical messengers that affect and regulate activity of the cellular mechanisms and metabolic function of organs. If these glands are dysfunctional, many hormonal problems can result. Glands must work together in harmony to restore equilibrium, balance, and to maintain a steady healthy state within our bodies.

This system, in close combination with the nervous system, helps sustain our internal environment. Endocrine tissues and glands are distributed throughout the body, and these include the adrenals, pituitary, thyroid, and sex glands.

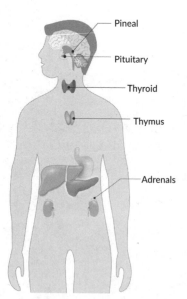

- Pineal
- Pituitary
- Thyroid
- Thymus
- Adrenals

There is an armory of herbs in nature's apothecary that promote glandular health, helping to regulate overall hormonal balance.

Glandular Tonics

Herbal tonics and botanical compounds exert a regulatory effect on the production of hormones. Herbal medicines help feed and renew the glands, helping to revitalize and bring each system back into a state of harmony, thus helping the body's inherent ability to heal itself.

Adrenal Glands

There are two adrenal glands, one above each kidney. These glands regulate metabolism, maintain fluid balance, and produce adrenaline that prepares the body for "fight or flight." The stresses of modern life can exhaust the adrenals, causing imbalance and adrenal fatigue. If our energies are exhausted, these glands will need the support of an herbal booster. The following herbs can tone the adrenals, stimulate, or relax them.

Borage (Borago officinalis)—Starflower

Originating from the Middle East, this herb is an age-old remedy and was used by medieval physicians to induce perspiration in fever victims. It has been an important herbal medicine since ancient times, and it was mentioned in *Culpeper's Complete Herbal*. Arab physicians in medieval Spain used borage to reduce fevers.

Borage was believed to have mood-altering powers, possibly due to its rich potassium content—a mineral that is quickly used up during stress. Borage is also known as "starflower," due to its star-shaped flowers. The oil that is extracted from the seeds of this herb is used to balance female hormones. The active properties of borage support the adrenal glands and they are also useful for the nervous system. Borage is easy to grow in an herb garden, and raw borage leaves can be added to salads and in infusions. It is available as borage oil or starflower seed oil capsules from holistic pharmacies and health shops.

Licorice Root (Glycyrrihiza glaba)—Adrenal Tonic

The medicinal use of this valuable plant stretches back 3,000 years and it is one of the most widely used in traditional Chinese medicine. The sweet tasting root supports the adrenal glands, due to its similar action to the hormone cortisol. Its tonic effect helps strengthen and tone the adrenals, promoting healthy function. It has a stimulating and regulating effect on the production of hormones, especially during periods of ill health and nervous stress.

This root has many benefits, one of them being to slow down the breakdown of adrenal hormones, which are usually in overdrive during stressful periods, and helps them to stay in balance. Licorice's adrenal-like effect is due to compounds that are similar to those produced by the adrenal cortex, and this makes this herb a useful alternative to steroid drugs in auto-immune disorders. This makes licorice an anti-allergenic, helping to dampen down an over-active immune system. It is available from health stores as capsules, tablets, tinctures, or herbal teas.

> **Warning:** If you are on any steroid drugs for auto-immune disorders, do not stop your medication, and do not use licorice root without consulting your medical doctor.

Rosemary (Rosmarinus officialis)—Adrenal Stimulant

Rosemary is a familiar evergreen shrub that is associated with remembrance, friendship, and trust—a connection that goes back to mankind's earliest records. Useful for adrenal exhaustion, rosemary acts as a stimulant, increasing the production of adrenal hormones. It uplifts and invigorates energy, easing tiredness, sluggishness, and loss of vitality when the adrenals are fatigued after prolonged stress. It is a strong herb and is only taken as tea.

Rosemary is a substance known as a "bitter," which stimulates the action of the liver, helping anyone who is suffering from "liverish" conditions. This term would describe the feeling we call "under the weather" and lacking in energy. An invigorating rosemary tea first thing in the morning allows the body to flush out toxins, assisting the body's own elimination processes and helping the system feel cleansed. It is available as *tisanes* (French for tea), infusions (teas made by using one teaspoon of the herb to one cup of boiling water), and tinctures.

Vervain (Verbena officinalis)—Adrenal Relaxant

This plant was sacred to the Romans who spread it on Jupiter's altars. In the Christian era it was considered a "witch plant," probably because it was so mysteriously therapeutic! The Druid priests, who were well versed in herbalism, collected vervain when the Dog Star was seen in the heavens. Also known as verbena, this herb is an adrenal relaxant that inhibits the production of adrenal hormones, helping to promote relaxation and stress reduction.

Vervain is an excellent herb to use when the whole metabolism needs stimulating. A soothing nerve tonic and a nervous system strengthener, this herb is helpful during a particularly stressful time when irritability, agitation, and anxiety are difficult to control. It helps to balance mental and physical energies and is thought to improve nervous vitality. Vervain eases emotional tension and is useful to use in adrenal exhaustion, depression, and stress overload. It has an uplifting quality that eases debility and depression due to its restorative properties. Infusions and tinctures are available from health stores, or medicinal herbal extracts from professional herbalists.

Thyroid Gland

The thyroid gland secretes hormones that help regulate body metabolism and the maintenance of body weight. This gland controls the action of all physical processes in the body. When the thyroid is out of balance, health suffers in a number of ways. Thyroid imbalance produces either excessive or insufficient chemicals resulting in too much or too little thyroxine in the system. This important hormone is produced by the thyroid gland, and it is rich in iodine. Iodine is necessary for the formation of thyroxine, and some of this element is stored in the gland itself. For balanced thyroid function, various herbs can prove helpful.

Bladderwrack Kelp (Fucus vesiculosus)—Thyroid Balancer

In the 1st century AD, Pliny the Elder referred to the use of kelp in his *Natural History*, and even today, these seaweeds are popular in America and Europe. Several species of seaweed are sold as bladderwrack kelp. Nature's sea plants are salty and toning, but this cool-water vegetable is a natural source of iodine. Iodine helps to synthesize the hormone thyroxine, which is necessary for healthy energy levels, fluid balance, and general good health. These thyroid stabilizers can normalize an underactive or an overactive thyroid, stimulating under activity or slowing down over activity. Kelp is helpful for goiter, which is the enlargement of the thyroid gland due to iodine deficiency. Kelp tablets are available in health stores.

> **Please note:** Any thyroid problem needs a doctor's diagnosis because goiter is not always due to a lack of iodine; an enlarged thyroid could be the result of a tumor.

Lemon Balm (Melissa officinalis)—Honey Bee Herb

An ancient tonic herb, lemon balm originates from the eastern Mediterranean. The name *melissa* is Greek, meaning honey bee. Lemon balm is also known as "bee balm" due to its ability to attract these useful pollinators.

This lemon-scented herb inhibits thyroid function, and it is useful for a slightly overactive thyroid. Its therapeutic actions are sedative and antispasmodic. Calming nervous tension, lemon balm uplifts the spirits and helps to restore stability from nervous exhaustion and fatigue. Recommended for soothing relief from stress and anxiety, lemon balm relaxes the whole system and normalizes the thyroid gland. A restorative with sedative properties, this calming herb is a valuable natural remedy for emotional stress or lack of concentration. It is helpful in mild hyperthyroid (overactive) states, helping to calm an irregular heartbeat. A hot infusion of lemon balm provides warmth and nourishment, while a bedtime infusion relaxes, and calms tension and anxiety. It is available as infusions, tinctures, and extracts.

Pituitary Gland

Called the master gland, the pituitary produces hormones in response to messages sent from the brain. This influential gland secretes hormones that stimulate other glands to produce their own chemical messengers. The pituitary gland regulates blood pressure, growth, stimulation of uterine contractions during childbirth, breast milk production, thyroid function, and function of sex organs inn both males and females—to name few! Malfunction of the pituitary gland lies at the root of many hormonal problems. Reproductive problems stemming from hormonal imbalances may benefit from sage or chasteberry. Pituitary harmonizers can restore balance overall to the glandular system.

Sage (Salvia officinalis)—Herb of Wisdom

Since antiquity, sage has been considered a universal panacea, due to its many curative properties. An attractive garden plant, sage grows best in sunny places. Red sage contains plant estrogens and it is used medicinally by women who suffer from irregular and painful periods. The volatile oils in sage are known to affect the pituitary gland, which confirms the long-standing use of this herb as a female tonic. Its fortifying and stimulating properties have long been recognized by traditional healers.

The pituitary produces several hormones, including those that stimulate the female ovaries, and others that control the menstrual cycle. During their reproductive life, women can suffer when hormones become unbalanced. Sage is used by women during various phases of life, and it is particularly useful during menopause to reduce hot flashes and to balance female hormones. It is popular with menopausal women who value its effective treatment of uncomfortable hot flashes. Sage is available as tablets, capsules, or infusions.

Chasteberry (Verbenaceae)—Vitex Agnus Castus

This herb is a deciduous aromatic shrub that is native to southern Europe. Used traditionally to balance the functions of the pituitary gland, thus helping to normalize the secretion of female sex hormones, *agnus castus* acts on the anterior pituitary, restoring stability to female hormones.

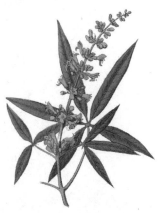

The pituitary gland sends out chemical messengers to regulate hormone stability, but sometimes these hormones become imbalanced and the use of this herb can be helpful in restoring balance, alleviating painful periods and related conditions. It is a natural remedy for premenstrual problems such as irritability, breast tenderness, water retention, headaches, acne,

Chasteberry

and heavy menstrual bleeding. It should be taken daily for three monthly cycles to obtain the full benefits.

Chasteberry is also a popular herb used for its harmonizing action on the entire endocrine system. It works well in combination with sage as a restorative gland tonic and it is available as tablets, capsules, or as a tincture.

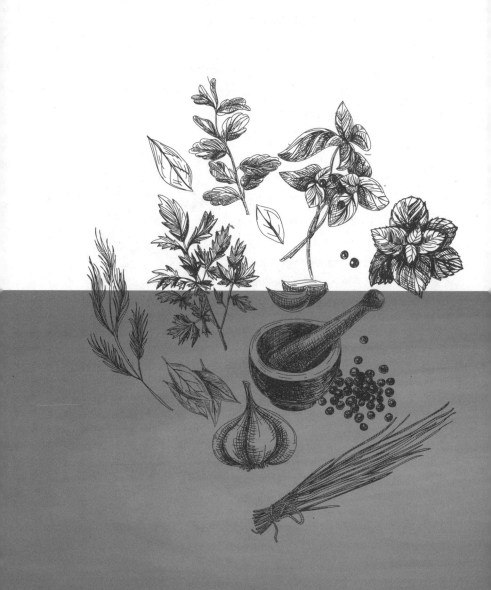

The Lymphatic System

10

*"Vitality & beauty are gifts of nature for those
who live according to its laws"*
—Leonardo Da Vinci

A network of vessels or lymph channels is the fundamental core of the immune system, and this network parallels the blood circulatory system. Lymph is a slow moving watery fluid that circulates around the body, picking up debris and cellular waste. Unlike the circulatory system, there is no equivalent of the heart to pump the lymphatic fluid around the body, so it requires massage, exercise, and skin stimulation to keep it moving. The body relies on the lymph system to drain away toxins. For good lymphatic functioning, you need to keep lymph moving so that it can clear your body of toxicity and the build-up of cellular debris that clogs the tissues. A healthy functioning lymphatic system that is free of waste on a cellular level is the key to health and healing. Traditional herbalism places great emphasis on purifying the bloodstream and the lymphatic system. Addressing problems in these two systems is a prerequisite to curing any other problem in any other body system.

Circulating lymph and white blood cells are important players in the body's first line of defense. There are specialized areas along the vessels of this system that create the various cells that the body uses to defend itself, including delivering immunity-providing white cells when needed. The immune system has the enormous task of protecting us against the onslaught of organisms that cause disease. When lymph is circulating freely, it is easier to stay healthy. When the lymphatic system is clogged with metabolic waste, the body's cells cannot absorb nutrients. This system plays an important role during a detox. Poor circulation and cellulite are signs of a poorly functioning lymphatic system. Herbs that purify are known as "alternatives," and these herbal cleansing agents help detoxify the lymph system, clearing it when it becomes overloaded and acidic, restoring it to a pure state.

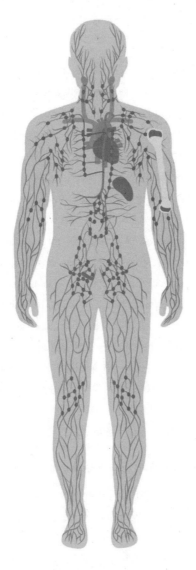

The lymphatic system

Echinacea—Lymphatic Cleanser

This herb is one of the most widely used blood cleansers in traditional herbalism. Echinacea's therapeutic benefits for seasonal ailments have been mentioned, but what is not widely known are its lymphatic cleansing and detoxifying abilities. This herb is a very effective herbal detoxifier for the circulatory, lymphatic, and respiratory system. Healing traditions place a high priority on protecting the body against forces that deplete its disease fighting capabilities, and cleansing the lymphatic system is believed to help keep all the body systems working well. Lymph is a major route for transporting nutrients throughout the body from the liver, and this herb is ideal for liver cleansing. When the lymphatic system is healthy and functioning well it can generally detoxify and eliminate most cellular wastes, but when it is sluggish and toxic, enlisting the help of a lymphatic cleansing herb will help the body cleanse and detoxify body tissues.

Decoctions, tinctures, or tablets (or echinacea tea if preferred) can be used to help clear cellular debris from the lymphatic system. Taken for short periods of time, this herb's cleansing properties can help keep this system healthy.

Cleavers (Galium aparine)—Blood Purifier

This common wild plant is a potent lymphatic tonic and is useful for cleansing the lymphatic system. It is used in herbal medicine for shrinking swollen lymph glands after a bout of infection. In traditional folk medicine, this herb is known as a blood purifier, acting through the lymphatic system. Gently cleansing and flushing out toxins, cleavers is used to detoxify the blood and to give a boost to the body's cleansing mechanisms. This herb is an effective diuretic used to purify the urinary tract of metabolic waste after an episode of cystitis (urinary tract infection). A lymphatic alternative, detoxifier, astringent, and harmonizer, this is a good herb for anyone who has experienced the discomfort of recurrent cystitis, or for those just interested in cleansing and purifying the body during different seasons of the year. Infusions and tinctures may only be available from herbal practitioners.

Red Clover (Trifolium pratense)—Lymphatic Activator

Traditional herbalism classifies this herb as hot and dry, and in medieval times these red flowers were thought to signify its blood cleansing properties. Red clover is also an important herb for cleansing lymph, and it has the ability to detoxify this system, promote body tissue renewal, and purify the blood. Working on the lymph, this herb has been found to activate the immune system by removing toxic congestion. This adds credence to its use by traditional herbalists who used it to treat tuberculosis.

In chronic toxic conditions, skin and glandular problems are linked to auto-intoxication, which is the process of the body poisoning itself with toxic residues, due to the eliminatory channels being laden and choked up with unhealthy waste. If these poisonous deposits are not removed, they will be reabsorbed into the bloodstream, further impacting health. Red clover can purify the lymphatic system, promoting health and restoring balance. This herb can be taken as a tea for a mild cleanse since the nutrients are easy to assimilate in tea form.

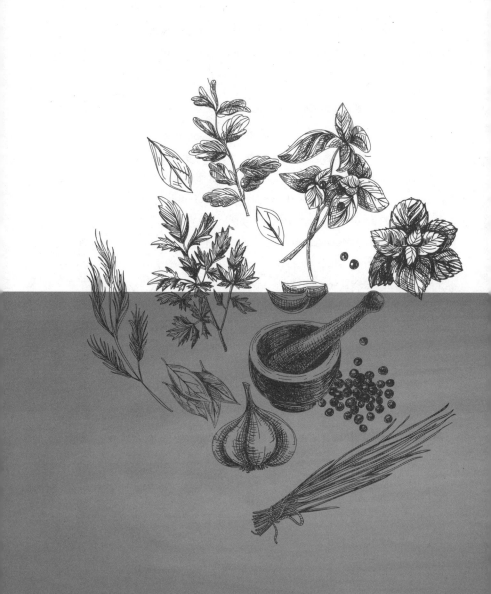

The
Muscular
System

11

*"The art of healing comes from
nature, not the physician."*
—Paracelsus

The muscular system provides the means by which the body carries out all forms of movement. The body's muscles cover bones and form flesh. Interior muscles, such as the diaphragm, divide the trunk into the chest and abdomen, and the muscles that form the walls of the organs, the heart, the alimentary canal, and so on, all come under this system. There are many problems that can affect the muscles, and nature has provided many herbs that help to ease muscular ailments, usually in the form of cleansing herbs that remove toxic wastes that may be lodged in the tissues. Common complaints include pain, stiffness, sprains, and swelling in the muscles and joints. These problems can develop into arthritis, so keeping this system healthy and flexible is important as people get older. There is a choice of various herbs that help in chronic conditions that afflict the muscular system.

Celery Seed (Apium graveolens)—Ancient Medicine

This traditional ancient medicine grows wild in marshy places. Also commonly known as "garden celery," it is widely cultivated. It contains flavonoids, antioxidants, and it has diuretic properties. Its therapeutic actions were well known among Roman and Greek civilizations, and today it is used in India by Ayurvedic doctors for rheumatoid symptoms, and it is also used in Chinese medicine.

Celery seed has gained popularity in the West as a musculo-skeletal pain reliever, nerve restorative, and relaxer. Celery seed supports a healthy inflammatory response and exerts a beneficial influence on kidney health, which is important to overall vitality. Celery seed has an alkaline reaction on the blood and is therefore a good detox remedy, helping the kidneys to clear wastes, especially the salts known as urates, which are inclined to accumulate

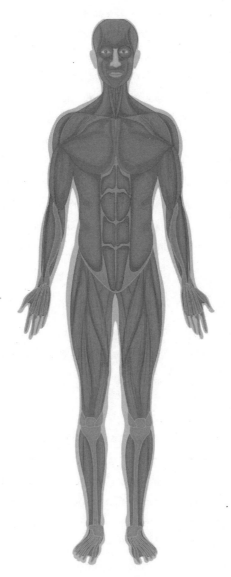

The muscular system

in joints causing stiffness, inflammation, and pain. Celery seed is also used for muscle cramps and spasms. It can be beneficial in the treatment of rheumatoid arthritis.

The diuretic action of celery seed extract is good for the painful inflammatory condition called gout, which is a disorder caused by the accumulation of uric acid in the blood, which causes a build-up of uric acid crystals in the big toe joint, as well as other joints in the legs, feet, hands, and arms. Gout is excruciatingly painful and disabling.

A green drink made from fresh, raw celery prepared in a juice extractor is a powerful cleanser of uric acid crystals, and celery seed tea is purifying and useful for a detox. It teams up well with willow bark.

Cramp bark (Viburnum opulus)—Natural Anti-spasmodic

This native shrub from the eastern United States has white, snowball-like flowers. The bark is gathered and used as an herbal medicine. As the name suggests, this herb is a powerful herbal agent that has anti-spasmodic properties and is used to relieve muscular tension and cramps. It has many therapeutic uses, especially for easing menstrual cramps and alleviating lower back pain. Its remarkable ability to relax muscular tension and spasm is attributed to its natural mineral content, which includes calcium, magnesium, and potassium—minerals that are well known for the beneficial effect they exert on muscle and nerve function. Cramp bark can also be used for relieving painful leg cramps and muscle twinges.

A good herbal muscle relaxant formula would be a combination of cramp bark with scullcap and valerian, but this may only be available from a professional herbalist.

Devil's Claw (Harpagophytum procumens)—Devil Root

This South African creeping plant grows in the Kalahari desert, and it has small spiny fruits that resemble hooked horns, and it is this that has given the devil's claw its name. The tubers possess anti-inflammatory, anti-rheumatic, and pain-killing properties. This herb has been used by African Sangomas and Inyangas (healers) for thousands of years. Sometimes called devil root, it has been shown to help ease backache, to increase suppleness and flexibility, and to improve mobility in the back and neck. Rheumatic or muscular pain has also been lessened by the devil's claw. Due to its anti-inflammatory properties and its muscle relaxing action, devil's claw is very beneficial for the relief of muscular problems resulting from sports injuries. It is available as tablets and capsules from health stores and holistic pharmacies.

Willow Bark (Salix alba)—Herbal Aspirin

Growing in damp, shady areas by European rivers, willow contains flavonoids and tannins. Known as an herbal aspirin, as far back as 400 BC Hippocrates prescribed willow bark infusions to relieve fevers and joint inflammation. In 1838, chemists identified the active ingredient, "salicylic acid," in the bark of willows, laying the foundation for the world's most famous medication, which we today know as aspirin.

This analgesic pain reducer is good for mild, inflammatory rheumatic states, painful muscles and joints, gout, rheumatoid arthritis, and backache. It has anti-spasmodic actions helpful for treating lower back pain and it is available as tablets, capsules, and as a tea.

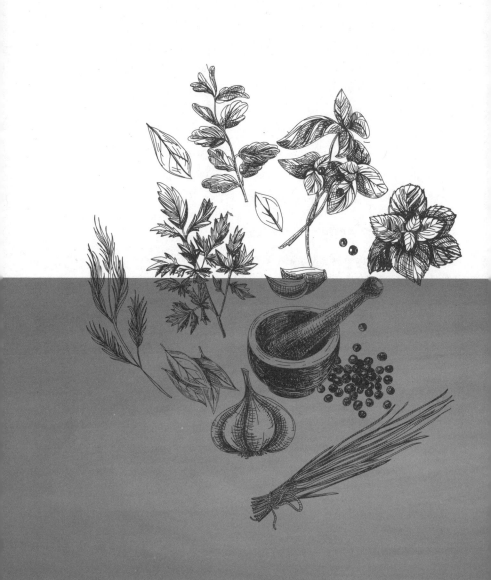

The Nervous System

12

*"He who is of a calm & happy nature
will hardly feel the pressure of age."*

—Plato

The nervous system provides the means by which we can respond to stimuli, and it delivers a system of communication between the brain and all parts of the body. Nerves can become depleted through stress, tension, depression, insomnia, and various other stimuli that cause nervous imbalance. To stay healthy the body must remain in balance, and while this is difficult in our stress-filled world, luckily there are natural remedies available that help us chill out. Migraine and tension headaches come under this nervous system umbrella, and various herbal medicines exist that will calm and balance jangled nerves and soothe nervous headaches.

The following herbs have been well tried and tested by herbalists and they have stood the test of time. Migraine headaches, nervous tension, insomnia, depression, lack of motivation, fatigue, and lack of desire are all problems that emanate from the delicate nervous system, but fortunately, the following herbs can revivify the whole nervous system.

Chamomile (Matricaria recutita/Anthemis nobilis)— Plant Physician

This sweet smelling herb was revered by the Ancient Egyptians for its curative powers and the astrologer priests dedicated it to the Sun. Today it is one of our most widely used herbs.

This small wild daisy has feathery leaves and a distinctive apple-like scent. Both German chamomile (*Matricaria recutita*) and Roman chamomile (*Anthemis nobilis*) are suitable for use. The difference between German and Roman chamomile is that the former is stronger, while the Roman type is less bitter. Both have a gentle soothing action. Both German and Roman chamomile are widely

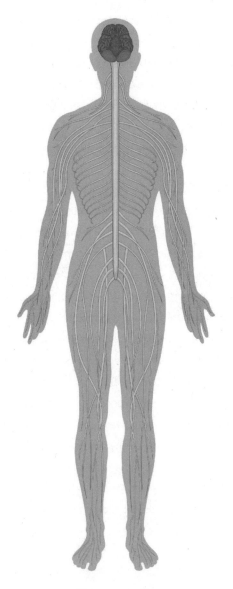

The nervous system

used and their actions are similar, so herbalists choose whichever they consider most appropriate for the problem they wish to treat.

This aromatic herb is a well-known relaxant and sleep inducer due to its sedative and curative properties. It reduces nerve excitability, helps calm and soothe nervous tension, hyperactivity, sleeplessness, and irritability. Honey can be added to sweeten chamomile tea to male it more palatable.

Lavender (Lavendula augustifolia)—Fragrant Relaxer

An evergreen woody shrub, lavender is a highly aromatic plant that grows well in the United States and Britain. Dedicated to the Greek goddess Hecate, goddess of the underworld, lavender was used by women who were preparing for childbirth because of its relaxing properties. Known as a tonic herb, lavender has a well-established tradition as a folk remedy.

Containing flavonoids and volatile oils, lavender is used often in aromatherapy as an inhalant for nervous headache, to relieve stress and panic, to calm and relax the mind, and for insomnia. Grown in the garden, lavender is a magnet for honey bees and butterflies. The dried flowers can be used to make a soothing lavender tea to drink during a migraine attack and to calm anxiety, nervous exhaustion, and tension headaches. Commercially bought lavender tea bags are available in health stores and some supermarkets. The essential oil is available through health stores and aromatherapists.

Rhodiola (Rodiola Rosea)—Golden Root

Growing in mountainous regions as far north as the Arctic, this root has a long history stretching all the way back to ancient

Greece. It was referred to as golden root because of its striking yellow flowers. It has a wide variety of uses, including use for long-term stress, as well as physical and mental fatigue. Used extensively in Russian folk medicine as an herbal tonic, this Arctic root is used today by herbal practitioners to aid their clients' physical and mental health when they are feeling low in energy. Rhodiola is also taken to relieve chronic fatigue, exhaustion, and anxiety.

Prolonged stress can deplete the body's defense mechanisms and rhodiola is thought to strengthen the immune system due to its adaptogenic properties. Adaptogens increase the body's resistance, normalize body functions, and restore balance. Rhodiola enhances stamina, improving tolerance to stress.

Oats (Avena sativa)—Nerve Tonic

Oats are a foodstuff that have nourishing and restoring properties. Prescribed by herbalists for centuries to treat depression and nervous tension, oat extract is well known as a stimulating nerve tonic that is used for mental fatigue and anxiety. It also helps to promote restful sleep. When eaten regularly, oats help the individual to recover from exhaustion and general debility. Oats, with their health-giving properties, assist the nervous system by restoring the hormonal balance.

Avena sativa contains many steroid-like molecules that tone a debilitated nervous system. These chemicals help balance the hormone testosterone in both men and women. Testosterone is the primary sex-drive hormone in both sexes, which may account for the phrase "sowing your wild oats"! Oats are a powerful brain and nerve restorative, combatting nervous exhaustion and strain, and they are used to support over-stressed nerves. Oats restore the glandular systems of the body, and they are very rich in nutrients. Oat extract is a useful tonic for debilitated nervous conditions. It can be used in the form of a nutrient cereal (porridge or oatmeal) or as oat extract tincture. Oats are contraindicated for those who are gluten intolerant.

Olive leaf (Olea europaea)—Tree of Life

Olive trees grow in warmer climates, and the Mediterranean area is most usually associated with the olive tree. Cultivated for thousands of years, the health-promoting properties of olive leaf were recognized by many ancient cultures. The Goddess Athena was reputed to have planted the first olive tree, and in Greek culture, the olive branch symbolized peace. The Ancient Egyptians believed that olive leaf was a symbol of heavenly power.

Used to help with a wide variety of ailments, the active ingredient is oleuropein. Olive leaf has powerful anti-bacterial and anti-viral properties, and it is used to relieve the nerve pain of shingles, owing to its anti-inflammatory actions. It also acts as an antioxidant. Shingles is caused by a reactivation of the chicken pox virus (*Herpes zoster*), which is present since childhood in anyone who caught the virus when young. *H. zoster* is an acute inflammatory viral infection of one or more spinal nerves or of the largest cranial nerve and it can appear again later on in life. The pain is intense because of nerve involvement—and as anyone who has suffered from it knows, there is no pain like nerve pain. Shingles tends to flare up when a person feels run down, but this nasty virus can erupt when the immune system is weakened by poor diet, infection, stressful situations, or old age. Olive leaf tea has been found helpful for this debilitating condition.

Valerian (Valeriana officinalis)—Nerve Soother

Valerian has been widely used since antiquity; the Ancient Greeks treated many ailments using valerian. It has been an important herbal remedy in Ayurvedic and traditional Chinese medicine for thousands of years. During the First World War, valerian was used to treat shell shock, and during the Second World War it was taken to ease the stress of continual bombing raids.

One of nature's most calming herbs, this powerful nervine promotes relaxation. Valerian's roots have a strongly unpleasant musky smell, a smell reminiscent of sweaty old socks! Today this herb's calming and tranquilizing actions are well known, and it continues to be in popular use as an herbal sedative, which is used to ease psychological stress. It is effective as a natural alternative to over-dependence on prescribed drugs (particularly tranquilizers), helping relieve tension, emotional strain, edginess, and nervous exhaustion—and it is non-addictive.

People suffering from sleep disturbances find that valerian offers an alternative way of getting a good night's sleep. This nerve relaxant's sedative and hypnotic action also provide mild pain relief during an attack of shingles. It is available as tablets, capsules, tinctures, and extracts, and valerian combines well with skullcap.

St. John's Wort (Hypericum perforatum)—Sunshine Herb

Growing wild along grassy banks and roadsides throughout Europe and the United States, this herb had a reputation as a protector against evil spirits. It was named after St. John the Baptist, as it was traditionally collected on his feast day, which is June 24th.

An ancient cure-all, St. John's wort is now popularly used as a nerve tonic. This species of *Hypericum* is easy to identify due to the many perforations that can be seen as dots when a leaf is held up to the light. Often referred to as the sunshine herb because of its attractive bright yellow flowers, this herb is used to calm nervous tension, anxiety, irritability, and depressed mood. Research has indicated that the chemical in the brain responsible for maintaining mood balance is serotonin, a neurotransmitter that is involved in many functions including the regulation of emotion and behavior; a deficit of this brain chemical leads to depression. St. John's wort appears to acts as a serotonin balancer, and many people who have used this herb for low mood and a depression have derived benefit.

An infused oil made using St. John's wort can be used to treat neuralgia (nerve pain) which is caused by inflammation of the nerve fibers. Warmed up and massaged along the area of the pain, this oil is very therapeutic. Today this herb is taken for mild anxiety, depression, and seasonal affective disorder. It is helpful for emotional problems experienced during menopause, it is effective in moderate depression. St. John's wort is a natural anti-depressant and a course of three to four weeks is recommended in order to feel the benefit of this herb's mood lifting properties.

Warning: If, after several weeks, you find no relief from depressive symptoms, you must consult a medical doctor.

Skullcap (Scutellaria lateriflora)—Stress Buster

This bitter nervine had a reputation in folk medicine as a cure for hydrophobia (rabies) and is known in America as mad-dog! It is helpful for any disease of the nervous system, and is effective for tense, nervy headaches, anxiety, and stress. Skullcap's relaxing properties can also help balance disturbed sleep patterns. The name itself is descriptive. It is derived from its shape, which resembles a skullcap.

A widely used nerve tonic, its cooling properties are helpful for the treatment of an over worried mind, helping to relieve tension and migraine headaches. Inducing calmness, and of value if suffering from disturbed sleep, this supportive nervine can also help with mental exhaustion if you have been working too hard for too long, or have been under prolonged stress.

Feverfew (Tanacetum parthenium)—Headache Reliever

This herb belongs to the same family as chamomile, and it has a pungent camphor-like smell. Growing in wastelands throughout the United States and in central and southern Europe and Britain, this herb's leaves have been used therapeutically to alleviate the severity and frequency of migraine. A cooling, bitter herb it was once used to treat fever—hence its name. Due to its anti-inflammatory action, it can also be used in cases of swelling and pain from arthritis. Today people buy this very popular over the counter herb to relieve debilitating headaches and migraines. A good pain reliever, feverfew relaxes spasms and dilates blood vessels. It is best to take it as soon as a migraine starts, as feverfew is less effective if the migraine has already developed. If grown in an herb garden this plant is highly aromatic and easy to grow. It can be taken as tablets, capsules, or in the form of fresh leaves.

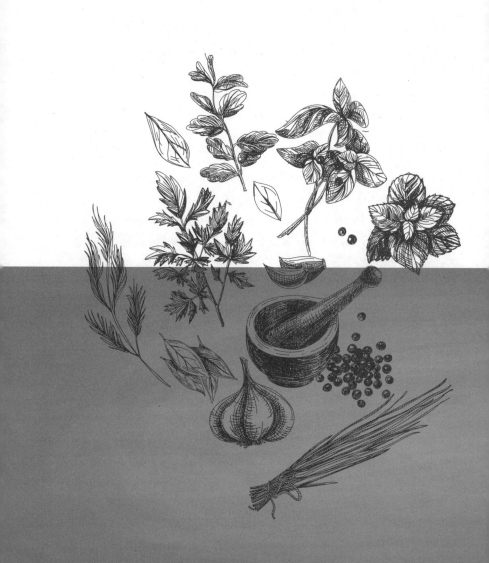

The Respiratory System

13

"Nature attacks the disease with whatever help she can muster."

—Paracelsus

The organs involved in breathing include the nose, mouth, larynx, and lungs. Air is drawn into and out of the lungs during which time oxygen is absorbed into the bloodstream. Oxygen is distributed from the circulating blood into the tissues in every part of the body, and carbon dioxide is removed from the blood and carried back to the lungs and expelled. The respiratory system is particularly vulnerable to chest infections, congestion, colds, bronchitis, and asthma. It is a system that needs care especially if there is a genetic weakness in this area. The cleansing actions of specific herbs encourage healthy respiratory health while supporting the lungs' natural detoxification process.

Mullein (Verbascum thapsus)—Lung Protector

Warning: If you are asthmatic, do not use this herb if you use inhalers.

This herb has been used as an alternative medicine for thousands of years and is a traditional all-round respiratory remedy. Legend had it that witches used mullein—which is also known as the candlewick plant—to make wicks for the candles and lamps that they used during rituals.

Mullein is used to support healthy lung function, and is recommended by herbalists as a lung tonic. Its actions are anti-catarrhal, soothing, and expectorant, removing sticky phlegm and relieving congestion. Its mild sedative properties help troublesome coughs, soothing lungs, and restoring health. In chronic respiratory conditions such as bronchitis and asthma, the saponin content of mullein helps loosen sticky mucus and stimulate expectoration.

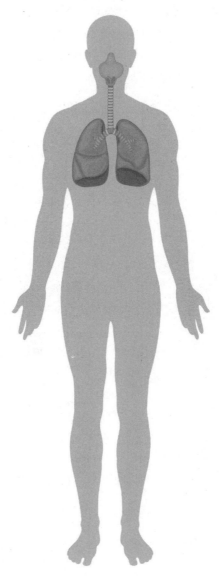

The respiratory system

Mullein soothes the entire respiratory system, pushing energies outward with a strong upward motion. Mullein is also a lymphatic cleanser. Mullein oil is available as an external herbal medicine for various ear troubles.

Marshmallow (Althaea officinalis)—Marsh Herb

Grown throughout Europe, marshmallow is well known in traditional herbalism. The Latin name *Althaea* is from the Greek, 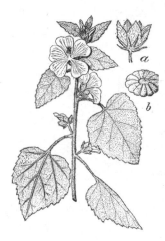 *altho*, meaning "to cure." Its demulcent action works as a soothing relaxant for respiratory ailments and supports the healing of hot/dry conditions. It helps moisten inflamed mucous membranes, acting as a good expectorant for unproductive, tickly coughs, bronchitis, and pleurisy. A traditional herbal remedy in Europe, the parts used are roots, leaf, and flower. Soothing and protecting irritated mucous membranes, its sticky consistency mimics the body's own mucus, helping reduce discomfort and inflammation. Found in cough syrups due to its anti-catarrhal, anti-tussive (against coughs) actions, marshmallow helps ease coughs by calming the cough receptors in bronchial and respiratory conditions. I

Thyme (thymus vulgaris)—Herb of Courage

Thyme is an old favorite for respiratory problems and it is still used today for the treatment of lung congestion and bronchitis due to its antiviral and antibiotic properties. Stimulating the immune system, this healing herb helps fight off colds, easing catarrh and troublesome coughs.

Thyme has a warm, uplifting fragrance with a pungent taste and a drying action. Native to the Mediterranean, thyme was burned as a sacrifice to the gods by the ancient Greeks who believed it inspired courage and bravery. In the solar temples of Asclepius, the God of Healing, thyme was used as an incense, and the oil used for fumigation against infectious diseases. A favorite of Greek physicians, thyme was used to treat infected wounds and snakebites. Thyme has long been known for its preservative and antiseptic qualities. In Ancient Egypt thyme was used in embalming fluid.

Thymol and carvacol are powerful antiseptics which are strongly germicidal, and these are responsible for thyme's medicinal properties. During the First World War, the oil was used to fight yellow fever in wounded soldiers who were brought back from the battlefield. It was also used as a hospital disinfectant.

Thyme is a tonic, stimulant, and pectoral (good for the chest) helping treat flu, coughs, fever as well as aches and pains. Acting as an antispasmodic, thyme is used in cough mixture compounds to soothe bronchial coughs. A good blood purifier, it filters toxins from the blood helping the healing process.

As a tea or gargle it is therapeutic for colds that have got a grip. Thyme's expectorant qualities expel stubborn bronchial phlegm, helping to loosen a dry aggravating cough. In traditional Chinese and Ayurvedic medicine, body energies are believed to be hot, cold, or damp. Thyme is said to direct hot energy outward emitting inner heat (yang energy) toward the outer areas of the body, moving the energies of respiratory infections outward to promote healing.

This is available as lozenges, cough syrups, and tinctures for chest tightness and coughs. Home-made teas using fresh or dried thyme can be brewed by boiling two tablespoons in 4 cups of water. Drinking this tea throughout the day will help soothe an inflamed respiratory tract.

Pelargonium (Pelargonium sidoides)—African Healer

Pelargonium is a natural antibiotic that is used in South Africa by traditional healers. Known by its African name of Umckaloabo it has been used for thousands of years by the people of the Basuto, Xhosa, Mfenfi, and Zulu tribes. In the West, *pelargonium* is known as rose geranium. Valued for its action on infections of the upper respiratory tract, coughs, ear, nose, and throat it is noted, for its ability to encourage rapid recovery from colds, flu, and chest infections.

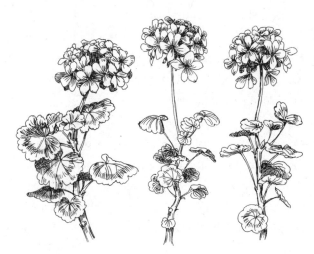

Pelargonium is used because of its anti-viral, anti-bacterial properties to treat bronchitis, respiratory infections and flu. Science has accepted that *Pelargonium sidoides* is effective in alleviating the common cold, which is something that traditional healers have known for thousands of years. If you have caught a cold or flu, or develop a chest infection, usually these infections tend to migrate downward into the respiratory tract, so taking a pelargonium extract can help stop bacteria and viruses from attaching to cell membranes and thus prevent them from multiplying. This herb is worth trying as soon as soon as you feel a cold coming on. If you come into contact with people who have flu, take some pelargonium tablets so that you will not succumb. Keeping a stock of *Pelargonium sidoides* during winter makes sense. You can buy tablets, syrups, and extracts from health stores.

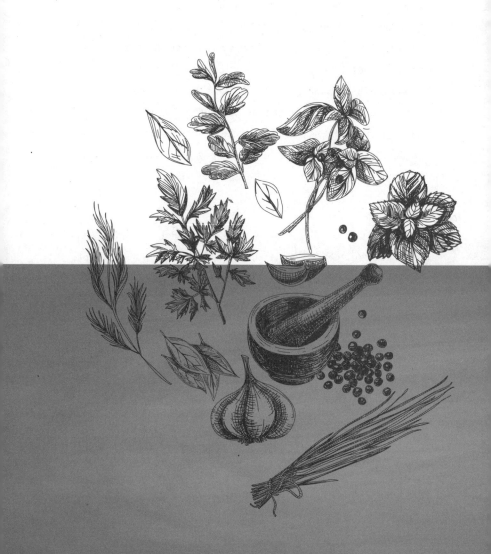

The Reproductive System

14

"Nature is a manifestation of Spirit."
—Ralph Waldo Emerson

This chapter will address the reproductive systems of both men and women. Each system is prone to its own unique problems and disorders, primarily tied to levels of hormones and hormone imbalance. Although both sexes can suffer from low libido, and men from erectile dysfunction, a component of these problems can often be psychological, and not necessary due to a disorder of the reproductive system. Therefore, this chapter will only focus on the physical/hormonal aspects of this system.

Women

The reproductive system lies in and below the pelvic cavity, and in women this area can be subject to many problems from puberty until menopause. These problems include pre-menstrual tension, heavy and painful periods, endometriosis, thrush, menopausal symptoms, and infertility, nature's garden provides herbs to help with these conditions.

Chasteberry (Verbenaceae) Vitex agnus castus— Hormone Balancer

Medieval monks used this herb to help them stay celibate in their sheltered monastic life, hence the name "chaste" berry. Today *agnus castus* is popular as a valuable herb for treating women's hormonal imbalances. The active ingredients of this herb act on the pituitary gland, which I previously mentioned in the chapter on the glandular system. The pituitary gland produces hormones in response to chemical messages sent to it from the brain during a woman's fertile years. In cases of infertility, this herb can increase the chances of conception as long as there are no structural problems involved. This is due to the fact that *agnus castus* keeps prolactin (involved in stimulating lactation) in check. The ability to decrease mildly elevated prolactin levels may benefit some, but not all, infertile women, as it depends upon the root cause of the infertility.

It is also helpful for women who suffer from breast tenderness associated with premenstrual syndrome. It can be taken for a few months, at least three, to gain its benefits. Like all hormone-balancing herbs it does not act instantaneously.

During menopause, when many women suffer hormonal imbalances, *agnus castus* can help alleviate some of the uncomfortable menopausal symptoms. Premenstrual tension, irritability, feelings of being bloated, and fluid retention will also benefit from a course of *agnus castus*. Excessive menstrual flow, menstrual cramps, and post-birth control pill imbalance can all be helped. It works well in conjunction with black cohosh.

Black Cohosh (Cimicifuga racemosa)— *Natural Estrogen*

Black cohosh is a perennial member of the buttercup family. For more than a hundred years, this herb has been known as useful natural medicine for women, and was used to induce labor. Cohosh is a Native American word meaning "rough" as the root of this plant is gnarled and twisted.

This herb has been well-documented as a natural alternative to hormone replacement therapy (HRT). In 1876 this North American herb was sold by Lydia Pinkham as a patent remedy for menstrual complaints. During menopause, the female hormones are disrupted, and this is one of the underlying reasons that women experience many unpleasant menopausal symptoms. Containing estrogenic substances, this herb is useful in conditions of estrogen deficiency. Rich in phytoestrogen, this herb is effective for reducing the discomfort of hot flashes, night sweats, depression, anxiety, and mood swings, which are symptoms that are often experienced during menopause. Plant estrogens are gentle estrogen mimics without the side effects of synthetic HRT.

Dong quai (Angelica archangelica)—Hormone Balancer

Also known as Chinese angelica, this herb is very popular in the Far East for women's problems. A common garden plant, *angelica* means "angel plant," a name that comes from its reputed powers against poison and plague.

This herb of angels comes into flower around Archangel Michael's feast day, hence its name. Its wide ranging action covers a number of female disorders, and it is commonly used to achieve hormonal balance during menopause. Chinese herbalists believe that dong quai keeps the uterus healthy by regulating the menstrual cycle, widening blood vessels, and increasing blood flow to various organs. Dong quai is taken for pre-menstrual tension, menstrual irregularities, menstrual cramps, and menopausal hot flashes. Chinese herbalists use the dried root as a uterine tonic, and it works well with chasteberry (*Vitex agnus castus*).

Red Clover (Trifolium pratense)—Natural Estrogen

The blood cleansing properties of this herb have already been mentioned in the chapter on the lymphatic system. Considered to be hot and dry in Chinese medicine, this herb is described as having yang energy, which is active and fiery.

Red clover's phytoestrogen compounds, rich in genistein, include a full spectrum of the isoflavones. Red clover's estrogenic actions help the sudden estrogen lows experienced during menopause, and can be used as an alternative form of hormone replacement therapy to relieve menopausal symptoms.

This herb can help ease many of the uncomfortable symptoms experienced during this normal life transition. It can also be used to address other female problems such as fibroids, endometriosis, and pelvic inflammatory disease (PID). It combines well with black cohosh.

Men

This system lies below the pelvic cavity, and is prone to various disorders during a man's life, including low sperm count, infertility, and prostate problems. The prostate gland lies immediately below the bladder. Prostate disorders are common in later years, and there are a number of helpful herbs that can be used to keep this gland healthy.

Saw Palmetto (Seronoa repens)—Prostate Healer

Growing wild in the southern United States, this small scrubby palm tree gets its name from the spiny saw-toothed stems. With a lifespan of over 700 years, it can resist insect infestation, fire, and drought. The red-brown-black berries hold the secret to its medicinal properties and healing powers. Native Americans used saw palmetto to treat sexual dysfunction and urinary tract disorders. Early colonists noticed that when saw palmetto was fed to their domesticated animals, their health and vitality improved, so this led them to use the fruits of the plant as a tonic. It was not until the 1990s that saw palmetto became popular for the relief of symptoms of an enlarged prostate.

Saw palmetto supports prostate health, toning and strengthening the male reproductive system. The medicinal benefits of this herb are well recognized and extracts of this plant are now an accepted treatment for benign prostatic enlargement, which can affect men of fifty and older. How does it work? It seems to reduce the absorption of abnormally high levels of two male hormones in prostate tissue, reducing inflammation and swelling. These actions help relieve the bladder obstruction that is experienced with benign prostatic enlargement, thus improving urinary flow. Its immune boosting and anti-bacterial properties may also prevent prostate and urinary tract infections. Rich in fatty acids and sterols, this herb is an effective general tonic for the male reproductive system.

Note: Any problems related to the prostate should be reported to a medical doctor and properly diagnosed in order to exclude anything serious, such as prostate cancer.

Pumpkin Seed Extract (Curcubita pepo)—Pumpkin Power

In ancient China, the pumpkin was known as "Emperor of the Garden" and it was seen as a symbol of good health. Pumpkin seeds are a rich source of a steroid-like substance called phytosterol, which counteracts hormonal changes that take place in the body of older men. Pumpkin seeds and oil are taken for their well-established nutritional benefits. The common pumpkin seed has been studied for its beneficial effect on the prostate gland, and has long been valued as a natural food for men's health.

Pumpkin seeds inhibit benign prostate enlargement. The high zinc and amino acid content of pumpkinseed oil is beneficial for the prostate. Pumpkinseed oil extract has shown benefits in reducing inflammation and other prostate symptoms, and to enhance bladder performance. Pumpkin seed oil is a helpful supplement for men to take for the proper functioning of the prostate gland and for prevention of future problems.

Pumpkin seeds can alleviate some infertility problems, as they supply beneficial zinc and amino acids that may be lacking in our modern diet. Pumpkin seed oil capsules are also "heart-healthy" as they contain plant sterols. Pumpkin seed oil comes in capsules or as loose pumpkin seeds and these work well with saw palmetto.

Pygeum (Pygeum Africanum)—African Bark

This is the bark of an evergreen tree that is found in Africa. For centuries, traditional African healers have used the bark of the pygeum tree to treat prostate problems. It works well with other herbs that are beneficial for prostate complaints. Pygeum works best with early benign prostatic hypertrophy (BPH), infertility, and impotence associated with BPH or inflammation of the prostate. It lowers levels of inflammatory compounds in the prostate, and is effective in reducing prostate enlargement. Its beneficial effects on the prostate gland are increased when taken in conjunction with saw palmetto.

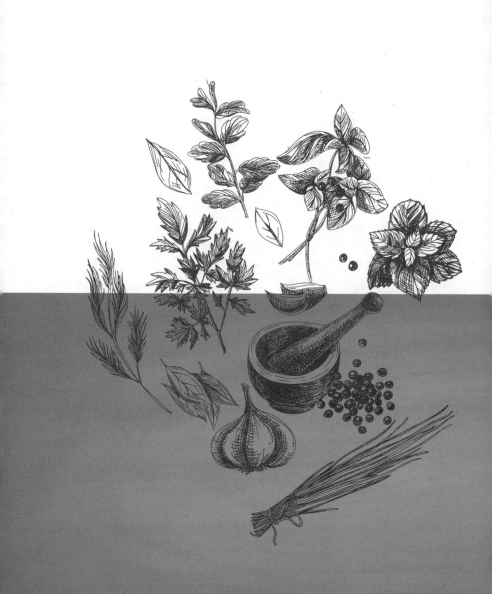

The Skeletal System

15

"Nature is man's healer."
—Deepak Chopra, *Quantum Healing*

The skeletal system forms the framework of the body, giving support, shape, and protection to all other parts of the body. The bones give form, rigidity and locomotion to the body, and they also serve as an incubator for red blood cells. Keeping this system healthy will help to prevent or alleviate many problems that are connected with the body's bone structure.

The skeletal system can be prone to a number of agonizing conditions such as arthritis, osteoporosis, and lack of mobility.

Rheumatoid arthritis is a chronic inflammatory illness where the immune system attacks the joints and other body parts. Osteoporosis, which is also known as brittle bones, also comes under this heading. This affects older people of both sexes; it is crippling, painful, and deforming, and the bone thinning aspect of this leads to many spontaneous fractures. There are a number of self-care steps that can be taken to help ameliorate the discomfort of these problems and these may help prevent the bones and joints from deteriorating further. These conditions usually take a long time to manifest, and herbal remedies are not an instant solution. They generally act slowly, and their effect is cumulative over time. The benefits can take weeks or even months to become evident, but it is worth waiting for as the risk of side effects from these herbs is usually low.

Boswellia (Boswellia serrata)—Indian Herbal Remedy

This traditional Indian medicine is sourced from the resin found in the bark of frankincense trees. Boswellia has long been highly prized for its ability to help with inflammatory conditions, and helps inhibit inflammation and builds up worn cartilage. It has

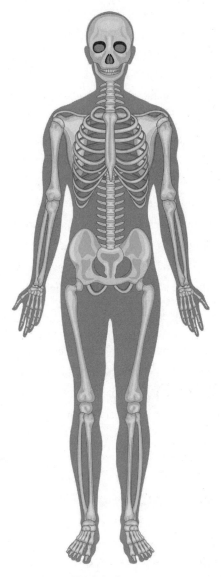

The skeletal system

been shown to hinder inflammatory chemical reactions in painful joints. This herb can treat varied conditions, but its anti-inflammatory properties have proved valuable in the treatment of arthritic pain. Boswellia is becoming a commonly used herbal medicine for stiff joint problems, and research has demonstrated its effectiveness and safety.

In rheumatoid arthritis, a particularly painful auto-immune disease, boswellia has been shown to reduce joint swelling, provide pain relief, increase mobility, reduce morning stiffness, and improve quality of life. Low back pain, soft tissue rheumatism, gout, fibrositis (pain and tension over the fibrous tissue of muscles and joints), may also respond positively to this Indian tree resin. Tablets containing standardized boswellic acid can be found in health stores and through Ayurvedic herbalists.

Devil's Claw (Harpagophytum procumbens)—Devil Root

We have already met the devil root in the chapter on the muscular system, but another of its talents is its use in easing joint pain and creating flexibility. The part used for this application comes from secondary roots or tubers. Traditional herbalists prefer the secondary tuber of the plant, as it has high concentrations of the beneficial components that help with arthritic problems. These compounds have anti-inflammatory properties and are helpful in many musculoskeletal problems.

Devil's claw is used in cases of arthritis and rheumatic conditions and as a complementary treatment for backache. Studies have shown extracts of this herb to be effective in relieving arthritic knee and hip pain. Gout is a form of arthritis, and the devil's claw has been shown to be beneficial in this very painful condition. It helps to remove uric acid from the body (this is a natural by-product of digestion) and it has also been demonstrated to have analgesic properties.

Taken by athletes to relieve tendon and muscle pain, it is beneficial in osteoarthritis and fibromyalgia, which is a neurologic disorder that is a common cause of chronic musculoskeletal pain and fatigue. Symptoms include generalized aches, and stiffness with tenderness on certain muscle points. It can be taken in tablet form, which are available in health stores.

Ginger (Zingiber officinale)—Joint Soother

Yet again we meet this remarkable herb with its heartening warming qualities—this time for joint relief. Osteoarthritis is a degenerative disease that affects the joints, causing pain and loss of mobility; it is usually the result of wear and tear on the cartilage of a joint and it is often age-related. Ginger has been used in traditional Chinese medicine and Ayurveda for the beneficial effects it has on the body, helping ease pain on worn joints. It was considered the king of tonics by Chinese and Indian herbalists. Its warming yang energies and circulatory action help joint mobility, thus relieving joint pain.

Ginger, one of nature's most multi-purpose and valued herbs, has been found to inhibit the formation of inflammatory chemicals that lead to joint pain. As we age, a lack of suppleness in the joints becomes more evident as the joints gradually lose lubrication and function. Because of ginger's warming action, it helps mobility and promotes flexibility. It has also shown promise in the treatment of rheumatoid arthritis, an auto-immune disease that is difficult to treat due to its inflammatory action.

Fresh ginger root is available in supermarkets, and capsules, tablets, tinctures, and infusions are available in most health stores.

Turmeric (Curcuma longa)—Spice of Life

Turmeric is a yellow spice native to South East India and is a main ingredient of curry powder. This yellow-flowered plant belongs to the ginger family, and in Indian and Chinese medicine it has been used for thousands of years.

Tumeric has been found to have a potent anti-inflammatory substance, curcumin, which has been proven to help in the debilitating disease of rheumatoid arthritis. Effective in the treatment of arthritic pain, tumeric's active curcuminoids reduce discomfort and swelling. Curcumin has been shown to have the ability to suppress the release of inflammatory chemicals that cause early morning joint swelling and stiffness. It has also been shown to be as effective as cortisone or phenylbutazone in models of acute inflammation.

Tumeric can be taken to ease the ache of sciatica, which usually is due to a problem in the lower back where the sciatic nerve becomes pinched and causes pain. Useful as a pain reliever, this herb can be used for arthritic discomfort, sports injuries, whiplash, and fibromyalgia.

It takes a concentrated supplement of turmeric to achieve its anti-inflammatory effect. A sprinkling of this spice in cooking is not enough to reap its benefits. Tablets and tinctures are available in health stores and the powder is sometimes available in supermarkets.

Meadowsweet (Filipendula ulmaria)—
Queen of the Meadow

This herb is a stout perennial of the rose family, and it is often called the "Queen of the Meadow." It grows in damp places and has a long history as a herbal analgesic and pain reliever in inflammatory conditions. The anti-inflammatory property is due to its salicylic compounds, which the body converts to salicylic acid, subsequently synthesized into the common pain killer that is now called aspirin. It has mild anti-inflammatory and anti-rheumatic activity and can bring relief to sore, stiff joints. This herb helps relieve the discomfort of rheumatic aches and pains and facilitates the removal of acidic wastes that accumulate in the joints. Meadowsweet is a prostaglandin inhibitor. Prostaglandins are inflammatory chemicals that are involved in pain and tenderness, and meadowsweet's analgesic action helps relieve the pain of swollen joints, arthritis, and rheumatism. Its cleansing properties helping clear acid wastes from the muscles.

It is available as infusions or tinctures, and it may only be available from qualified herbalists.

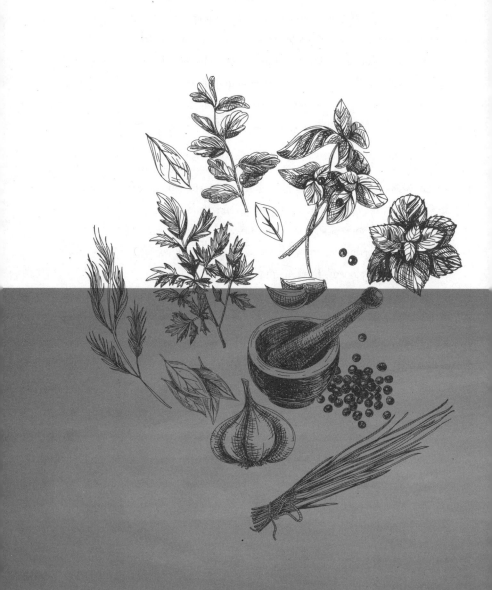

The
Skin and Eyes

16

"Archangel Michael, after Adam's fall,
anointed his eyes with eyebright."
—Milton, *Paradise Lost*

Through our skin and eyes we literally wear our health on the outside of our bodies. They are the two most obvious health systems of which we are aware every day. The eyes are actually part of the nervous system, which was discussed in chapter 12. But because of their uniquely outward placement, like the skin, I will discuss them here.

The Skin

The skin is a dynamic living organ that responds to internal imbalances. It is the largest organ of the body, and it eliminates wastes that cannot be removed through the normal internal channels. Skin problems are often a sign that the body is trying to excrete poisons and wastes through the pores. Known in natural medicine as the third kidney, the skin is prone to many problems. Traditional herbalism relates skin blemishes and acne to blood impurities and circulating toxins, and we use herbs that are described as "alternatives" to cleanse the system. Throwing off stored waste with the help of herbal cleansers improves the skin and makes it look younger.

Acne, eczema, psoriasis are all skin problems that do not always respond well to conventional medicine; those medicines may be effective in the short term but they can also be suppressive to other body systems. Blood purifying herbal remedies have been shown to improve skin problems.

Burdock Root (Arctium lappa)—Detox Herb

Burdock is an important purifying remedy in traditional herbalism and Chinese medicine. A detoxifying herb, burdock is useful in the treatment of acne, boils, and eczema, along with psoriasis and skin infections. This herb eliminates waste products in chronic skin conditions. Burdock can be used in any health problem that requires detoxification and waste clearance. It has a stimulating action that helps release toxins from the cells, and has antibiotic properties. In skin disorders there may be an initial worsening of the condition, a skin flare up, which is a healing crisis during which the body attempts to reinstate balance.

Psoriasis is an abnormal condition in which extra skin cells build up rapidly on the surface of the skin. It differs from other skin problems since it is an auto-immune disease, and the causes of this disease are not fully known.

Skin problems can be intractable; in treating difficult skin conditions one needs patience before results can be seen. Using this blood cleanser may show benefits in skin conditions that have proven difficult up to now. It is available in tablets, tinctures, and decoctions, and it works well with dandelion or red clover, as these herbs counterbalance burdock's strong detoxifying actions.

Cleavers (Galium aparine)—Skin Cleanser

This weedy annual is also known as goose grass because geese love to eat it. It is a lymphatic cleanser with cooling properties and its detoxifying action makes it a good treatment for skin problems. Skin can accumulate years of toxic wastes, and cleavers exerts a strong influence on the lymphatics, producing an herbal cleanse when combined with burdock and/or dandelion. This is particularly useful for treating eczema and psoriasis. Use of this herb can help maintain healthy lymphatic functions, clearing the skin of accumulated wastes. It is available in tincture and infusions, although it may only be available via herbal practitioners.

Dandelion (Taraxacum officinale)—Gentle Purifier

Traditional herbalists have valued dandelion for its gentle blood cleansing action and for helping to clear toxic states involving skin problems. The condition of the skin is a reflection of the inner health of the body, and it is a good monitor of the general state of health. With the use of gentle cleansing herbs such as dandelion, chronic skin conditions resistant to mainstream medicine can be helped. Boils, acne, eczema, and psoriasis are distressing conditions, and the use of this common weed may prove useful in these difficult-to-treat skin troubles. Available as a tincture or infusion, but probably only from professional herbalists. Dandelion combines well with burdock.

Nettle leaf (Urtica dioica)—Blood Cleanser

This garden weed has many uses as a blood cleanser, and nettle is a good detox remedy. Due to its high flavonoid content, it is helpful for alleviating many types of skin conditions. Cleansing and anti-allergenic, nettle will help relieve many skin conditions, especially those that are itchy, inflamed, and uncomfortable, such as eczema, psoriasis, and rash. A rich source of trace elements, in particular silicon, makes nettle's whole body toning properties valuable in supporting skin tissue.

Using nettle infusions as a lotion can relieve inflamed skin, while tablets can be taken to cleanse the blood and detoxify a congested system. It is available in tablets, tinctures, and leaf infusions in health stores. For intractable skin problems, an herbal practitioner can design a specific mixture.

The Eyes

Bilberry (Vaccinium myrtillus)—Sight Saver

Bilberry is a shrubby perennial that grows in the woods and meadows of northern America and Europe. This herbal sight saver is used to maintain healthy vision, and it is believed to help prevent glaucoma, cataracts, and age-related macular degeneration. Its medicinal qualities derive from anthocyanosides—a class of powerful flavonoids—which are the plant's main components. These are potent antioxidants that help neutralize free radical damage to the cells. In particular, bilberry acts on the eye's micro-circulation, increasing oxygen and energy levels in the eye and strengthening eye tissue. Taken long term in tablet form, bilberry can act as a preventative, protecting against eye damage and vision problems that may develop with the aging process.

Eyebright (Euphrasia officinalis)—Eye Tonic

Eyebright has been traditionally used to heal eye afflictions, and for its tonic effect on the mucous membranes of the eye. Eyebright is also used for treating common problems of the eyelids (conjunctivitis) or pink eye. Eyebright's actions are toning, and this herb can be taken internally, as it is thought to relieve eye inflammation, dry up excess watering, and heal the surface of the eye. Eyebright is also taken to improve vision.

> **Note**: If your eye is infected, eyebright might have a soothing affect, but you must consult a medical doctor for treatment.

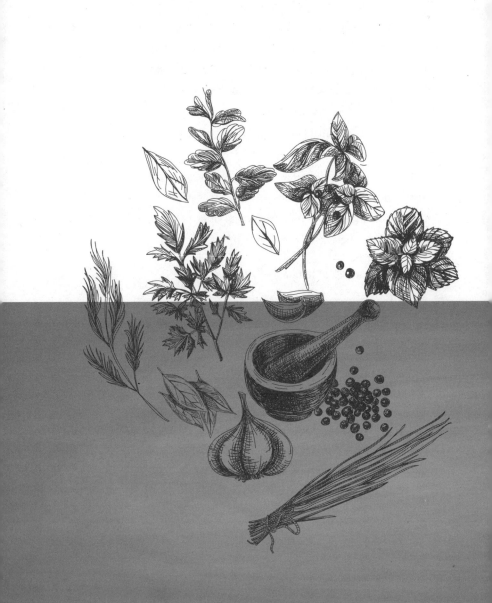

The
Urinary
System

17

"For medicine we used the herbs
of the fields and gardens."
—Jethro Kloss, *Back to Eden*

The urinary system lies in the abdominal and pelvic cavities, and performs the vital task of excreting body wastes, cleansing the body of cellular debris, and helping to maintain a constant internal environment. Diuretic herbs are used to help the kidneys in their important work of cleansing this system. Women suffer more urinary tract infections than men, mainly due to their physical anatomy, and there are various herbs that can help this system in the herbalist's armory.

Cranberry (Vaccinium macrocarpon)— Nature's Urinary Cure

Cranberry is an evergreen shrub that blooms in midsummer. Before they open fully, the delicate rose-tinted flowers resemble a crane's head and neck, hence the name. Early herbalists were familiar with this plant, as were Native American healers. Cranberry contains flavonoids and other natural compounds, and it has been found to help support a healthy urinary tract, prevent cystitis, and help maintain the natural pH balance in the bladder. Compounds in cranberry prevent harmful bacteria from sticking to the bladder walls.

Warning: Repeated attacks of cystitis are often indicative of pre-diabetes, so you should always avoid juice that has been sweetened with sugar or corn syrup.

Cystitis is a painful condition and cranberry's antibacterial and anti-inflammatory qualities reduce the inflammation and help clear infection from the urinary tract. Cranberry can be used on a regular basis to prevent cystitis if you are prone to this painful condition. It is available as an unsweetened juice, as tablets, and in powder form.

Cleavers (Galium aparine)—Urinary Cleanser

Another of this versatile herb's actions is its effectiveness a urinary antiseptic. Rich in chlorophyll and vitamin C, cleavers is an effective diuretic that clears bladder infections and cleanses the urinary tract. It may also help prevent kidney stones from forming. Infusions or tinctures are made up by professional herbalists only.

Marshmallow (Althaea officinalis)—Urinary Soother

This traditional European herb has been used by humans for thousands of years, and pollen from a species related to the marshmallow has been found in a 60,000 year old Neanderthal grave!

The medicinal component is mucilage, which soothes and calms the mucous membranes, both internally and externally. Taken internally, marshmallow leaf is used for its soothing action on the bladder and urinary tract, and it is used for mild cystitis. It helps alleviate irritations of the urinary tract. Tablets can be found in health stores as infusions or decoctions. It is also available from professional herbalists.

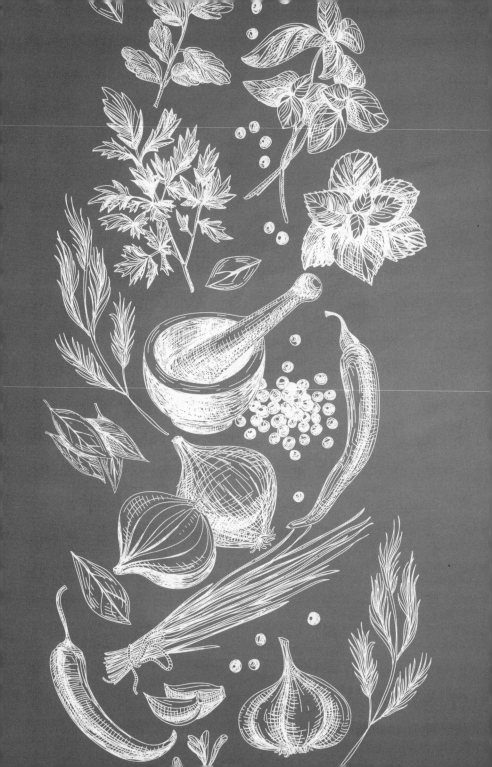

Part Three

HERBS
FOR
EVERYDAY
USE

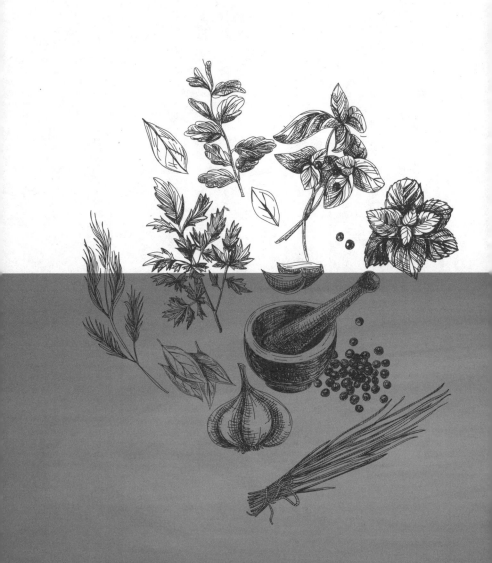

Herbal First Aid Kit

18

"In nature's perfect design nothing ever dies."
—Deepak Chopra, *Quantum Healing*

You can make a basic herbal first aid kit for your home and use it for various simple conditions. The following herbs are the must-have basics in you first aid kit. They are safe and effective herbs and ointments that cover most common ailments. These can either be found in most good health food stores or you can prepare them from herbs grown in your own herb garden. These home remedies can be used to treat minor problems such as colds, stings, bruises, sore throats, and headaches, and also prevent more acute problems from setting in.

Arnica (Arnica montana)

Widely used in herbal medicine, this herb is anti-inflammatory and analgesic (pain relieving) so it is useful for easing bruises and sprains it is also used for sports injuries. Available in tincture form, cream or gel.

Aloe Vera Gel (Aloe barbadensis)

Known in America as a "first aid plant," this is a useful addition to your herbal first aid kit. Applied topically, it is an excellent and effective gel to use for minor burns. Useful also for rashes, its soothing qualities and anti-inflammatory activity help repair damaged tissue. It soothes insect bites and stings.

Marigold (Calendula officinalis)

Calendula in cream or ointment form is healing for minor cuts, grazes, stings, and mild burns. Applied topically, it will soothe angry inflamed skin; taken as a tincture, it helps cleanse and detoxify the system. It can be used as an ointment or as a tincture.

Clove oil (Eugenia caryophylatta)

This oil is a strong antiseptic, and a useful addition to your home first aid kit. Dampen a cotton ball with clove oil and hold it against your teeth and gums to relieve the pain of toothache until you can get to see your dentist. DO NOT USE ON TEETHING BABIES.

Lavender oil (Lavendula augustifolia)

This all-round oil is used by aromatherapists for many physical conditions, and it is useful to relieve mild burns, insect bites, and bee stings.

Tea Tree Oil (Melalauca alternifolia)

This antiseptic oil should be in everyone's herbal first aid kit, as it is used for the treatment of minor wounds and fungal infections. Tea tree is anti-bacterial, anti-fungal and good to use as a germicide against virulent organisms. Check when buying Tea Tree oil that it is of sufficient potency and not blended with other oils.

Witch Hazel (Hamamelis virginiana)

Apply distilled witch hazel to sprains and strains to reduce swelling. You can also use it to clean wounds. Neat or diluted, it is soothing and cooling, with a spicy, pleasurable fragrance.

St. John's Wort oil (Hypericum perforatum)

Apply a poultice of warm St. John's Wort oil onto sprains or neuralgia. If a sprain gets worse after twenty-four hours, see your doctor in case there is an underlying broken bone. This oil will help dull the nerve pain of shingles and it will speed healing.

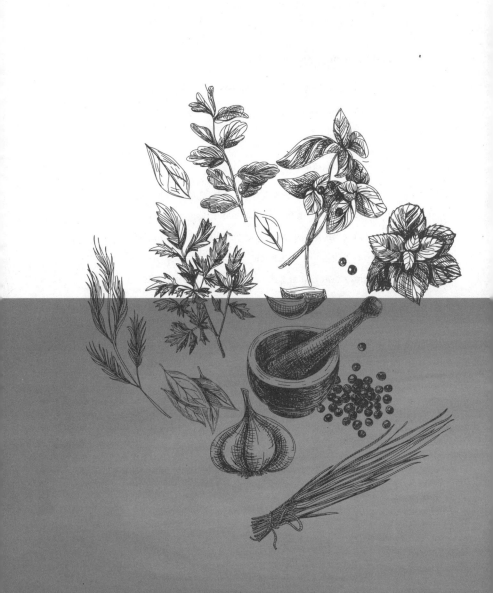

Health
from
the Hive

19

"The hives of bees being rubbed with leaves of
bawne causeth the bees to keep together."
—John Gerard, *The history of plants,* 1597

B elieved to be the Nectar of the Gods, honey was used in ancient times as a medicine and it is often still used as such today. Herbalists believed that honey was a potent healer, having observed its wound healing properties among its various other health benefits. It was also used as a heart tonic. Hippocrates, the "Father of Medicine," extolled the virtues of this "liquid gold" and recommended honey for healing ulcers. There is evidence that the use of honey has been around since as far back as 6000 BC. The therapeutic benefits of honey are mentioned in ancient Egyptian hieroglyphic writing, as well as in Asian and Chinese literature, dating back thousands of years. Honey also finds a mention in the sacred scriptures of both the Bible and the Koran. Records from 2000 BC show honey being mixed into pastes and applied to the skin after surgical procedures. Honey was also used for healing abscesses and boils.

Honey's active property is its hydrogen peroxide content, which is highly antibacterial. Unlike synthetically produced hydrogen peroxide, the natural form found in honey *only* destroys bacteria and it is completely harmless to healthy tissue. Thus honey has been used to treat a wide range of conditions ranging from burns to cataracts without damaging sensitive tissue.

Herbal Medicinal Honeys

Herbal medicinal honeys are made of raw honey because it contains many of the beneficial properties and enzymes of the plant from which the honey was derived. Those beneficial properties are often lost when honey is heated. Mass-produced honey does not have the medicinal qualities of raw unheated, untreated

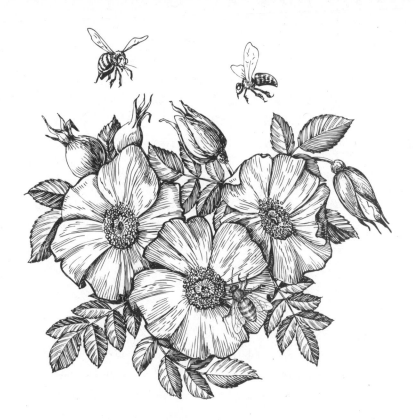

honey, and only raw honey will have the bioactive properties nec-essary for healing. Some of these honeys can be found in health shops or organic farm stands. One can make honey at home and then eat some every day, by adding it to herbal tea or whenever you need an energy boost.

Dandelion Honey

This is light-amber in color and has a strong flavor. Dandelions are essential for bees as they are a rich source of pollen and nectar. Wild dandelion honey has a tangy, rich flavor, and adds a delicious flavor to herb tea.

Eucalyptus Honey

This dark amber honey has a sweet clover-like taste. It is mainly found in independent health stores, and it is a good standby to have at home when winter is approaching. It is good to drink in herbal tea if you feel a sore throat coming on.

Heather Honey

Rich and dark, this honey is produced in the British Isles, but honey from heather that is grown in the Scottish Highlands differs from that which is produced in Britain, as the Scottish variety has a distinctive dark reddish brown color with a strong flavor.

Hymettus Honey

Called "Nectar of the Gods," this ancient honey has been produced for 3,000 years in the region of Mount Hymettus, which is to the south east of Athens in Greece. This honey derives from a special variety of an aromatic thyme that grows wild on Mount Ymitos. Considered one of the best high quality honeys, Hymettus has a rich, dark, smoky flavor and it can be used medicinally. Runny and tinged with flecks, its unmistakable aroma is redolent of the sharp woody fragrance of thyme. This delicious ancient honey is well worth a try.

All of these medicinal, herb-infused honeys can be taken throughout the winter by the teaspoon, or they can be added to a cup of warming herbal tea.

To make an herbal honey you need one cup of honey and two tablespoons of a chopped fresh herb of your choice. One tablespoon of a dried herb can be used, but a fresh herb's natural properties will be more potent. Pour the honey into a small sauce-pan and warm it over a low heat. Once it is warm but not hot, add the herb of your choice and stir it in.

Another method of making an herb-infused honey is to add an herb to a clean jar, pour the honey over the top, stir and close the jar with a tight fitting lid. Steep this for one to two weeks on a sunny windowsill, turning the jar over each day to redistribute the herbs. You can strain out the herbs or leave them in.

Manuka Honey—the Rolls Royce of Honeys

From New Zealand we have a very special honey that is known as Manuka. It is called "mono-floral" honey, which means the bees interact with only one species of flower, gathering pollen only from the Manuka bush to make this sticky, delicious honey. This honey is causing much excitement in the medical world.

The Manuka bush is unique to New Zealand. Research has shown that not all honeys are created equal, and Manuka appears to have powers far beyond other honeys. The Maori people have used the Manuka plant for medicinal purposes for centu-ries (*Manuka* means Tea Tree in Maori). They use the leaves of the Manuka plant to make an herbal drink when they need to lower a fever. The oil from the crushed leaves is also applied to wounds because of its antiseptic properties.

Clinical research has found Manuka honey effective in treat-ing a wide range of difficult to heal wounds, ranging from post-operative cancer and mastectomy lesions to amputation wounds and leg ulcers in diabetics and the elderly—it has a very strong anti-viral and anti-bacterial action. Mainstream medicine is turning to this ancient healing honey to deal with infected wounds that no longer respond to antibiotics. Researchers have found that the intractable bacteria, *helicobacter pylori*, can be effectively inhibited by Manuka honey when taken internally. *H. pylori* causes painful infection, and is associated with stomach ulcers. It can lead to stomach or bowel cancer.

This medicinal honey can also be used to calm the gastrointestinal tract, helping to reduce symptoms associated with the common problem of irritable bowel syndrome. The old folk remedy of drinking warm milk with honey for a good night's sleep has its roots in truth, as Manuka or any other unprocessed honey has analgesic properties that can help to soothe the mind and body, promoting restful sleep.

Manuka can be used to sooth sore throats, heal difficult skin infections, and as a general daily pick-me-up to prevent colds and flu. A few teaspoons of this nutrient rich honey in a daily warm herbal tea is an excellent way to avoid colds and flu during the winter season.

There are many strengths of Manuka available, so be sure to look for the UMF logo on the label (the unique Manuka factor) as this will guarantee you are getting the real product. The stronger the strength, the higher its therapeutic activity.

Pollen, Propolis, & Royal Jelly

Pollen, propolis, and royal jelly are three natural products from the hive that are great to use in helping to build stamina, vitality, and health. Royal jelly is the substance that comprises the queen bee's diet, enabling her to live for much longer than other bees.

Pollen—Nature's Energizer

The value of pollen has long been recognized by many indigenous cultures. While collecting nectar to make honey, bees gather pollen as their main protein food. Pollen contains protein, carbohydrates, fats, and a varied assortment of nutrients, and our ancestors recognized its therapeutic value. The New Zealand Maoris have eaten pollen for centuries, and they also used it to make pollen cakes. Linked to cultures that live to over a century, pollen is a super food that boasts a huge number of health benefits, and although I cannot guarantee that you will live for a century if you take this power-packed natural substance, it can certainly have an energizing and rejuvenating effect if taken on a regular basis. Heat-treated honey removes the pollen content, but tablets or granules are available from health stores. Modern day athletes take pollen to improve their endurance, while anyone who wants to be fit or to recover from some condition can benefit from pollen

Bee pollen taken prior to the start of the hay-fever season may help reduce the severity of allergic reactions. Bee pollen encourages the immune system to form antibodies against the allergic response. There are many pollen preparations in health stores and it is a matter of choice whether you take pollen granules that can be sprinkled on yogurt or breakfast cereals or in tablet form. The tablets should be taken on an empty stomach.

Propolis—Nature's Penicillin

Propolis comes from a Greek word that means "defender of the city." This material protects the colony from invasion, and it prevents the spread of infection. Used by the Ancient Egyptians, Romans, and Greeks for its healing benefits, today it is used to prevent or treat several medical disorders. The most active properties of propolis are compounds called flavonoids that contain anti-oxidants that are protective against cell damage. Propolis has been shown to kill viruses that man-made medicine has yet to find an effective remedy against.

Known for over 3,000 years as a natural health defense against infection, propolis can be used on a continual basis to maintain good health during the changing conditions brought by each season of the year. Liquid propolis has been shown to have anti-allergenic properties, and it can benefit allergy sufferers during spring and summer season. This substances has a remarkable capacity to stimulate the human immune system and to protect against bacterial and viral infections. It is available as tinctures, lozenges, tablets, or as liquid propolis, and as a throat spray.

Royal Jelly—Food Fit for a Queen

One of the most concentrated natural substances known to nature, this mysterious jelly is a unique nutrient-rich substance that is produced by worker bees for the nourishment of the queen bee. It is the glandular secretion produced by young female honeybees. The queen bee is fed a nutritious diet of royal jelly by her court of worker bees. She lives a long life and her sole biological function is to reproduce on a massive scale, by laying around 2,000 eggs a day. She is fed this wonderful nectar all her life; hence, royal jelly has a reputation of being an elixir of life. The only difference between the queen and the other bees is her diet.

Practitioners of folk medicine have used this rich substance as a tonic for hundreds of years, in particular in traditional Chinese medicine. This could be attributed to the fact that royal jelly is exceptionally rich in natural hormones, vitamins, and amino acids. Royal jelly can improve your well-being, boost your natural defenses, and help you adapt to the pressures and strains of daily life.

It can be found in your local health food store, but make sure that you buy a good quality, fresh royal jelly if you want to try this valuable food supplement, as the freeze-dried variety does not have the potency of the fresh one. A course of royal jelly will help you feel vitalized, it will increase your stamina, and it will promote energy, so it can be used as a tonic boost a couple of times a year. It is usually available in health stores in its fresh form.

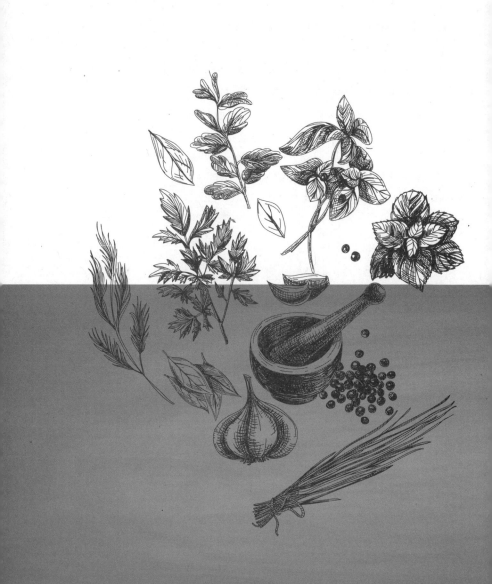

Herbal Elixirs 20

"There is tremendous power in reclaiming our health care."
—Aviva Romm, herbalist,
midwife and teacher

erbal elixirs are all-rounders that benefit every body system. They are fast acting energy boosters that are taken to enhance vitality, and to keep the body and mind healthy. Elixirs are also called decoctions. There are many herbal elixirs in the form of tinctures, tablets, syrups, and liquids in health food shops. Useful as an aid to recovery after illness when the body is still convalescing, they can help speed up the healing process. They are useful in post-viral fatigue when the body is still debilitated from fighting off a nasty viral or bacterial infection. Toning elixirs help to restore the body's energies.

Ginseng (Panax Ginseng)—Ancient Elixir

Panax ginseng exhibits a supporting effect on the immune system, and helps you recover from fatigue and weakness. This revitalizing fluid is made from the whole ginseng root, which provides more active ingredients than extracts, thus giving maximum effectiveness. In liquid form, ginseng is faster and better absorbed.

You can improve your health and vitality by taking ginseng for two or three weeks twice a year, just before the start of summer or winter. One dose (ampule) should be taken before breakfast every day over a two to three week period when you need extra energy or when trying to adapt to stressful situations. Take it in the morning on an empty stomach, either neat or in fruit juice. Liquid in premeasured ampules are available in health stores or from Chinese herbalists.

Guarana (Paullinia cupana)—Amazonian Vine

Guarana comes from the seeds of a woody Amazonian vine. The seeds are roasted and ground, and the powder is mixed with water and sugar to make it into a drink. The tribes of the Amazon basin drink this refreshing potion daily, and believe that it increases stamina and improves vitality. Its stimulating properties are due to a chemical called guaranine that acts like caffeine. Unlike caffeine in coffee, the stimulating properties of guarana are released slowly, thus improving mental alertness and supporting energy.

Guarana is an adaptogen that helps the body to maintain a proper stress response, and it can be used to boost energy or after a bout of illness. Athletes like to take this as a drink to make them more alert and to enhance their performance. It can be useful to take guarana as an energy boost a couple of times a year. It is available as tablets, drinks, and powder form, in health stores and most pharmacies.

Premium Fresh Royal Jelly—Ambrosia of the Gods

Royal jelly in solution can be taken in ten milliliter glass ampules. These ampules are available in higher doses in health stores and Chinese herbalist shops. In China, where the people have long understood the principles of natural balance and harmony, royal jelly drinks are used as an instant energy boost.

A ten milliliter ampule can be taken after a long journey to boost flagging energies, or at each transitional season to improve health and vitality, or before strenuous physical or mental activity. In its fresh state, this nutritious and powerful complex is one of nature's richest health foods, and it will help maintain overall good health. Boxes of ten milliliter (10 ml) ampules are available in health stores and from Chinese herbalists.

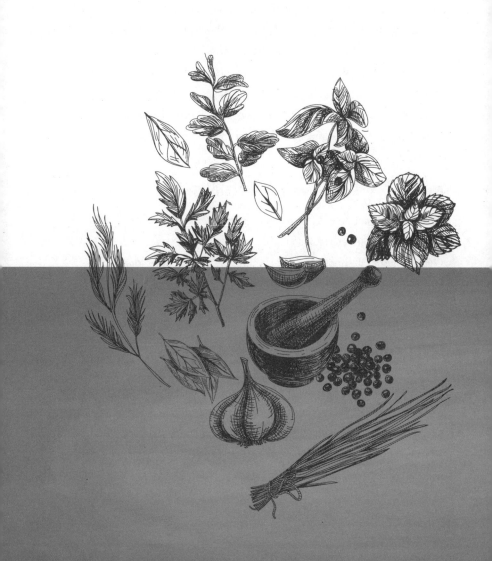

Anti-Aging and Tonic Herbs

21

*"Every man desires to live long
but no man would be old."*
—Jonathan Swift

There is no mythical fountain of youth, and alas, not even plants can halt the march of time. But . . . they can slow it down a bit; several plants contain youth-preserving phytochemicals. Traditional herbalists believe that the aging process begins when the body's energies become depleted over the passage of time. Evidence today suggests that a downward aging spiral is not as inevitable as was once believed, and many factors other than time are involved in the aging process. The aim is for youthful maturity and good health throughout life. Nature has provided some natural anti-agers and their therapeutic properties can be effective in keeping the body youthful and full of vitality.

Anti-Aging Herbs

The following herbs may help slow down the rate at which the body ages on a cellular level by strengthening the immune system and preventing oxidation caused by free radicals. Rejuvenating herbs help rebuild the body, increasing energy levels, stamina, and vigor.

Amla (Emblica officinalis)—Ayurvedic Rejuvenator

Ayurveda is the ancient holistic healing system of India that utilizes natural herbs, roots, and plants to promote harmony and well-being. Legend has it that over 3,000 years ago, nature revealed the secrets of the beneficial properties of each tree, plant, herb, root, and flower to the sage Dhanwantari during meditation. A number of these beneficial herbs are available in the West, and today Amla (Indian Gooseberry) can be purchased in health stores and from

Ayurvedic practitioners. Amla is a bitter due to its tannin content, but it is rich in vitamin C and other antioxidants that help prevent free radical damage.

Amla is recommended to be taken over a long period of time to replenish, rebuild, and invigorate the body's systems.

Echinacea (Echinacea angustifolia)—Skin Protector

This versatile herb may help slow down the aging process of the skin. This is believed to be due to echinacea's ability to block a destructive enzyme that breaks down collagen and elastin in the dermis. It is a potent immune booster that helps the body to resist infections. Regular use of this multi-purpose herb will help strengthen the immune system and it may help slow down the aging process.

Thyme (Thymus vulgaris)—Herb of Youth

The process of cellular protection has led to the idea that thyme can help deter aging that results from free radical damage. Renowned for its broad spectrum properties, this herb is believed to promote longevity. Thyme helps prevent the breakdown of essential fatty acids in the brain that are necessary to keep this vital organ young, so its reputation for promoting brain health and long life may be well deserved. If you grow this herb in your garden, pick the leaves when the herb is just going to flower, and add some to your salad dressings to keep old age at bay.

Thyme leaf tea can be made using fresh sprigs of thyme, and you can make an infusion in the same way you would make a pot of tea. This tea can also be used as a cosmetic, which, when cool, can be patted onto the skin to help the complexion.

Tonic Herbs

Tonic herbs are known as adaptogens or harmonizers. They help to tone the system when energies are depleted or to calm an over active system. The root part of the plant is most frequently used. These tonics can be used as a short course to revive flagging energies after winter, and whenever you need a boost.

Astragalus (Astragalus membranaceus)—Chinese Tonic

This traditional Chinese herb contains many compounds including flavonoids, amino acids, and trace minerals, and it is used as a tonic herb. Native to China, astragalus is one of the most popular herbs there, where it is used to boost energy levels and

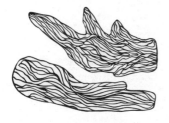

Astralagus

improve endurance. Known to be a potent immune stimulant that increases white blood cells production, astragalus improves stamina during exercise. Current herbal monographs indicate that this herbal root supports the activity of white blood cells, antibodies, and other protectors that the immune system mobilizes when defending the body against viruses and bacteria.

Taken as a vitality tonic a couple of times a year, this herb helps the body to adapt during seasonal changes, keeping the system in balance and fortifying natural defenses. A course taken as winter is approaching, is a good way of strengthening the body's resistance. It is available as capsules and tablets in health stores.

Ginseng (Panax ginseng)—Oriental Magician

Ginseng has been used as a tonic in Chinese nutrition for over 5,000 years. During the Han dynasty, the ruling Emperors allegedly ordered their subjects to search the mountains for this curiously shaped root, specimens of which were worth their weight in gold. Emperor Sen Nung stated in his *Pharmacopoeia of the Heavenly Husbandman*, around the 2nd century AD, that ginseng was a "king among herbs." The name means "Wonder of the World," and it is derived from the ancient Chinese "Jen Shen" meaning "man root," because it resembles an upright human figure. Warming, stimulating ginseng is a yang herb, its tonic

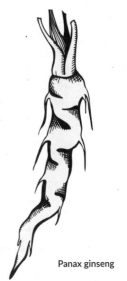

Panax ginseng

effects restoring equilibrium, vitality and balance. An Ancient Chinese text called the *Pen Ts'aos* represents 4,000 years of Chinese wisdom and medicinal knowledge; it notes ginseng's energy-promoting properties and its use as a general pick-me-up. Panax ginseng has also been called "touch-me-not" because of the plant's intimidating thorns. Panax comes from the Greek word "panacea," or cure-all.

There are many different types of ginseng; the North American varieties are milder than the Oriental types. The two most commonly used ginsengs are Korean and Siberian. The former is masculine and corresponds to yang (hot) active energy. It is said that one of the benefits of taking the Siberian variety (passive and cold in nature) is that it can help clarify thought and balance the emotions. According to herbalist Penelope Ody, "Siberian ginseng, traditionally feminine (yin), can be more suitable for women."

In the sophisticated Chinese healing system, this herb is used to balance chi, which is the life force that runs throughout the body's energy meridians. When taken for mood improvement, increased physical performance, and to relieve stress, it is considered to quiet the spirit and prolong life. Attributed to living more than a century, Chinese sages believed ginseng had a reputation for longevity. It is an adaptogen that acts as a tonic when energy is low and exerts a calming influence when energies are over active.

Added to its formidable reputation as a cure-all, ginseng has also been used for its aphrodisiac properties. No doubt its shape contributed to the belief that it was an Oriental Viagra! This potent healer can work its therapeutic magic throughout the body, helping maintain good health and restoring depleted energies. It can be taken in tablet or capsule form or as a tea, and it is available in health stores. Ginseng root is also available from Chinese herbalists.

Ashwagandha Root (Withania somnifera)—Indian Ginseng

Ashwagandha is used in Indian Ayurveda, a healing system called "The Science of Life and Longevity." This root is considered to be a vitality tonic. It is a popular Indian herb that is used to reduce stress and facilitate learning and memory. It has powerful antioxidant effects wherein it scavenges free radicals and removes them from the body, including the brain and other major organs. Described in ancient Ayurvedic medicinal texts as a health promoting energizer, this restorative root has been used in Ayurvedic medicine safely and effectively for centuries.

Ashwagandha's qualities help in the treatment of many health problems such as anxiety, stress, and depleted energy. During winter, when some people suffer from a dip in energy levels and low mood caused by lack of direct sunlight (SAD), this tonic herb can help boost energy, vitality, and improve mood.

Ashwagandha strengthens the nervous system and helps to calm it. It is relaxing and harmonizing, and it helps to improve the activity of the immune cells. The toning properties of this herb are helpful when there is a stress-related condition that needs calming down or strengthening, as in the case of exhaustion. It can help to treat the kinds of nervous weaknesses that we

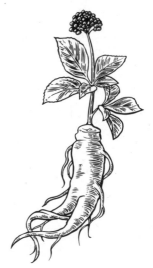

Ashwagandha (Indian ginseng)

are prone to in this fast-paced modern world. A good balancer of body and mind, aswagandha also helps support the immune system after a bout of illness, restoring it back onto an even keel.

Ashwagandha is similar to, but not the same as, Panax ginseng. Ashwagandha is capable of calming psychological stress by reducing activity in the central nervous system. Panax ginseng is more stimulating, and increases quickness in attentional-task performance. An overload of panax might make you feel anxious, whereas too much ashwagandha can potentially cause drowsiness.

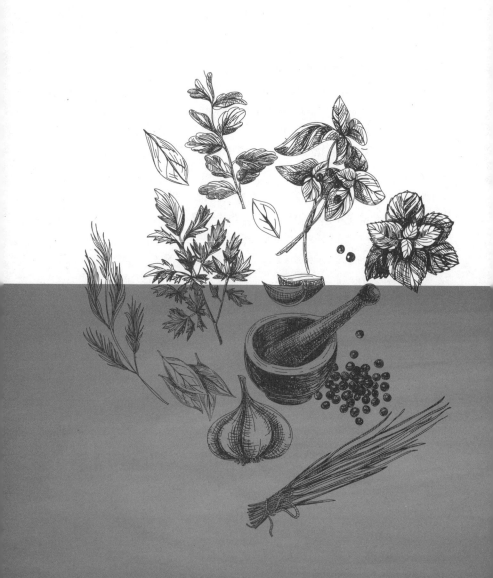

Aromatic
Herbal
Baths

22

"The way to health is to have an aromatic bath and a scented massage every day."
—Hippocrates

There is nothing more soothing than submerging yourself in a warm scented bath. Herbal baths provide healing benefits for mind, body, and spirit. They can relax you, energize you, and ease muscle tension and stiffness. Used therapeutically in ancient times, herbal baths were a well-known therapy. This idea is thousands of years old and rooted in the healing traditions of Ancient Egypt, Greece, and Rome.

Bath sachets made with dried scented flowers or essential plant oils can be used. Relaxing bath herbs include passionflower, chamomile, and verbena, while stimulating bath herbs include lavender, mint, rosemary, and pine. Healing herbs include yarrow, marigold, and comfrey. Put a handful of herbs into a little muslin pouch and hang it by a long loop onto the bathtub tap so that hot water flows through it as the bath water runs. Herbs release their therapeutic properties into the water, smoothing and soothing the skin, relaxing the nerves, and stimulating flagging energy. The herb pouch can be rubbed over the body and used like a gentle scented loofah.

Essential oils can also be used for a therapeutic bath soak. Aromatherapy is an age old therapy that uses concentrated oils extracted from plants, flowers, fruits, leaves, root and barks. They are nature's living plant essences. Bathing in fragrant waters is uplifting, and it will enhance your physical and emotional well-being. Run a bath, add three or four drops of essential oil, but be careful not to use too much because these oils are potent and may agitate sensitive skin. Then agitate the water and step in.

The choice of oil is up to you depending on the desired effect. Always look for 100 percent essential oil and make sure the oil is a good quality.

> **Note:** Essential oils are powerful, so mix a little with warm water and test on a small area of skin before plunging in.

There are calming oils for relaxation, relief of tension, and when you need to ease tired muscles and aching limbs. There are clarifying oils when your energies need stimulating, and balancing oils to restore your equilibrium. When you need a boost, an energizing oil would be appropriate. Last but not least there are oils that have such a wonderful aroma they give you an uplift improving your mood due to their heavenly fragrance. So why not soak away your worries after a tough day?

Use the following oils in your herbal bath for healing the spirit, mind, body, and emotions, for reinstating balance and for the maintenance of health and vitality.

Eucalyptus oil

Eucalyptus oil is cleansing, stimulating, and uplifting. The woody sweet scent of eucalyptus clears the head, helping to relieve mental sluggishness. This oil can help you breathe more easily, loosen stubborn chest and nasal mucus due to its expectorant properties, and it can rejuvenate the spirits. It belongs to the green family of oils.

Ginger oil

This fiery and fortifying oil has tonic properties calming nervous conditions. It blends well with orange oil for a warming winter bath, helping to ease coughs, colds, and everyday muscular aches and pains. It may be best to avoid this if you have sensitive skin. It belongs to the spicy family of oils.

Lavender oil

Lavender oil is a versatile, soothing, restorative with a soporific fragrance. With its analgesic properties, this oil is used to unwind and relax relieving all kinds of tension-related problems, balancing the nervous system, calming the nerve-endings of the body, aiding restful sleep and steadying emotions. It is a real stress buster. It belongs to the floral family of oils.

Orange oil

This orangey, zesty fragrance stimulates, revives, revitalizes, and awakens the senses. It is warm and cheering and is a good addition to a warming winter bath. It belongs to the citrus family of oils.

Peppermint oil

Peppermint oil refreshes, enlivens, and invigorates. The cool minty fresh fragrance elevates the spirits, refreshes the mind and perks up the senses. It belongs to the green family of oils.

Pine oil

Pine oil is sharp, fresh and stimulating, refreshing, and healing. In bath water this oil helps alleviate fatigue due to its invigorating action. A pine oil bath can also be very good for cystitis and other urinary problems due to its antiseptic properties. It belongs to the woody family of oils.

Rosemary oil

Widely used in the Middle East two thousand years ago, rosemary helps loosen tenacious chest and nasal mucus because of its expectorating qualities. It invigorates, energizes, and awakens a tired mind, easing everyday muscle aches and pains. Stimulating, warm, and penetrating, this essential oil is analgesic but not sedative. It belongs to the green family of oils.

Tea Tree oil

Tea tree oil is a powerful disinfectant with a strong medicinal aroma. This antiseptic oil from the Australian outback cleanses, purifies, and fights viral and fungal infections such as athlete's foot and ringworm. It belongs to the spicy family of oils.

Ylang Ylang oil

Exotically fragranced, ylang ylang's heavy, sweet, warming aroma creates a calm, sensual mood, and promotes a sense of well-being. It is perfect for pampering. It belongs to the floral family of oils.

Stimulating	Calming	Purifying
Eucalyptus	Ginger	Ylang ylang
Orange	Lavender	Tea Tree
Peppermint	Ylang ylang	Pine Oil
Pine		Ginger
Rosemary		Rosemary

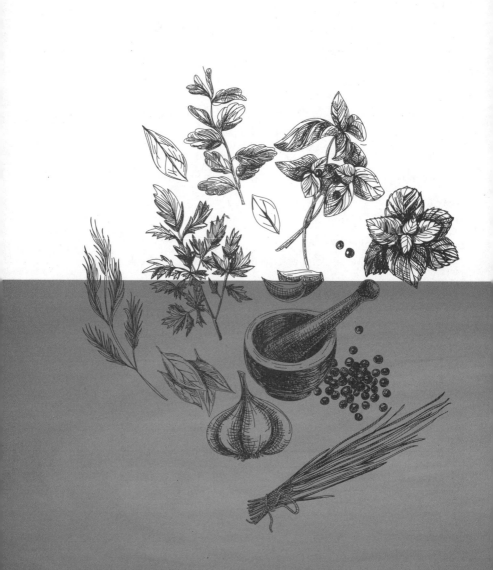

Herbal
Teas

23

"A day without tea is a day
without joy."
—Chinese Proverb

The first herbal tea was reputed to have been discovered by the Chinese Emperor Shen Nung. Legend has it that a gentle breeze blew some *Camellia sinensis* (tea bush) leaves into the Emperor's cauldron of water, and he enjoyed this brew so much that it started the trend of what was the world's first cup of tea! Whether this is true or not, teas have been enjoyed for hundreds of years and recently are enjoying a revival.

Since ancient times, tea drinking has been a ritual in Asian countries to keep the body in good health. In Japan's many tea houses, spiritual tea ceremonies are a tradition that are over three hundred years old. Green tea is said to have life-prolonging properties due to its anti-oxidant content. Japanese ancestors laid down the traditional philosophical system of Chado, or "Way of Tea," and Japanese spiritual tea ceremonies are performed by a ceremonial tea maker in order to help induce harmony, purity, peace, and tranquility.

Today we are once again discovering the therapeutic value of herbal teas. These teas are gaining popularity, with many varieties now easily available. If you want a change from conventional tea or coffee, herbal teas make a pleasant, healthful drink that doesn't contain caffeine, so they can be taken at any time of the day. Make them part of your healthy life style and you will soon become a fan when you experience their uplifting and healing properties.

Anyone with an herb garden can make a tea from leaves, flowers, bark, seeds, berries, or roots of certain herbs for medicinal purposes, or simply for the pleasure of drinking an herbal brew for its taste. If you don't grow your own herbs, a wide variety of commercial tea bags are now easily available from health shops or supermarkets. Herbal infusions (teas) can be sweetened with honey. They can also be livened up with cinnamon sticks and cloves for a spicy, warming drink.

Chamomile tea

Chamomile is one of the best known herb teas. For centuries chamomile tea has been used as a nerve sedative. If you are over-tired and weary, this tea's soporific qualities have a calming effect, soothing your nerves after a tiring day. This tea with a teaspoon of honey will help you to unwind before you go to bed, when your brain is exhausted and overactive. Chamomile's sleep-inducing action will help induce restful sleep. It is a wonderful way to relax at any time of the day.

Echinacea tea

Echinacea tea is often drunk during winter to help strengthen the immune system. Echinacea's powerful properties can improve resistance against colds and flu. This herb has a broad-range effect and can be used to alleviate a number of ailments including urinary tract infections, sore-throats, and bronchitis.

Ginger tea

With its pungent, warming taste, ginger is good for nausea, and for morning sickness during pregnancy. To treat motion sickness, either chew a fresh ginger root or eat some crystallized ginger. Yang in nature, it is great in colder months to get the circulation moving.

Ginseng tea

Ginseng tea has a rich earthy flavor and is good for an energy boost. The tonic effects of this tea are strong and have a whole-body effect, energizing all body systems. According to Jean Carper, "The Russians have conducted more than four hundred studies on a single ginseng; repeatedly they affirmed that people drinking Siberian ginseng tea appear healthier, feel better, withstand stress better, have more energy and concentrate better." The benefits of this energy-giving tea is something that Asian cultures have known for centuries!

Green tea

Tannins give this potent tea its sharp, astringent taste. Chinese herbalists recommend green tea to remove heat, due to its cooling properties. Green tea contains group of compounds called catechins, which are a type of polyphenol, plus high concentrations of antioxidants; attacking free radicals, green tea is a potential anti-carcinogenic. These compounds help liver function and have been shown to have powerful heart benefits. Because of its caffeine content, green tea would be too stimulating to be taken before bedtime. It can be enjoyed with a teaspoon of honey to take the edge off its sharp flavor.

Lemon Balm tea

This tea is made from a handful of fresh lemon balm leaves, and it makes a refreshing and restorative lemon-scented infusion. Cooling in nature, this herb is helpful to take as a tea to help ease tension and take the edge off mild depression and low mood.

Lemon balm inhibits thyroid function and it can be used for a slightly overactive thyroid, which may cause symptoms of anxiety.

Licorice tea

Licorice is a known stomach-settler and it is also good for colds, coughs, and sore throat relief. Licorice is an adrenal tonic, so this tea is good to take when energies are flagging. It tones the adrenals, thus helping to resist exhaustion.

Peppermint tea

One of today's most popular herb teas, peppermint is used as a digestive and to stimulate a depressed appetite. Its crisp refreshing flavor is cooling, and women who suffer from menstrual pains would also find a cup of peppermint tea helpful, as its antispasmodic properties help alleviate cramps. Peppermint makes a good after-dinner tea that settles digestion, and the minty refreshing taste of peppermint tea is soothing and effective during the cold and flu season.

Rosemary tea

This tea is made from the evergreen flowering rosemary shrub. Crush the green needle-like leaves and inhale the strong bracing herbal aroma. The penetrating vapor will help to clear your mind.

To make an aromatic tonic tea out of rosemary, pour some boiling water straight onto two or three sprigs of rosemary in a teapot. Infuse this for several minutes then strain and drink this invigorating and uplifting tea warm. It can help clear your head, and can be taken with honey if preferred. You could try this first thing in the morning to kick-start your day!